YOU, YOUR PARENT, AND THE NURSING HOME

YOU, YOUR PARENT, AND THE NURSING HOME

NANCY FOX

Prometheus Books
Buffalo, New York

Published 1986 by
Prometheus Books
700 E. Amherst Street, Buffalo, New York 14215

Copyright © 1986 by Nancy Fox

First published in 1982 by Geriatric Press, Inc., Bend, Oregon.

All rights reserved. No part of this publication may be reproduced, stored in a retrieval system, or transmitted, in any form or by any means, electronic, mechanical, photocopying, recording or otherwise, without the prior permission of the publisher.

Library of Congress Catalog Card No. 86-83887

ISBN 978-0-87975-317-7

To my husband, sociologist and Doctor of Philosophy, whose philosophy for years has been to support and encourage me in all my endeavors, and to my

Four sons, Robin, Phil, Sam, and Stephen, still young, but old enough to understand that the later years can be a challenge, a creative time of life, and to

Patricia O. Smylie, of Baton Rouge, Louisiana, whose invaluable suggestions for this book make her someone special in my professional and personal life, and to

All members of the Grand Generation—your parent in particular—those bearers of our heritage, in each of whom shines a spark of divinity.

Contents

	Preface: A Letter to You, the Family	9
1	Filling Beds—or Filling Needs?	13
2	Sizing Up and Selecting a Nursing Home	24
3	A Mighty Fortress, the Family	45
4	How to Diagnose the Doctor	53
5	Who Cares for Your Parent?	67
6	Is This Senility Necessary?	93
7	Think Therapy	102
8	When Mother Is "Difficult"	118
9	Sexuality at Any Age: Part of Being Human	125
10	For Your Parent, Life More Abundant	134
11	The Nursing Home Is What You Make It	144
12	When Your Parent Is Terminally Ill	157
	Concluding Message to You, the Caring Family	162
	Appendix	164

Guilt, depression, fear of censure—many emotions plague you, the family that has placed, or must soon place, a parent in an institution. How to cope? As an outsider, what is, or will be, your role? Have you any more "say" in what happens to your parent? Is the home you have chosen a good one, or is it a commercial depository?

How can you meet your parent's needs and still preserve your own life and other responsibilities?

Your questions are valid. You deserve forthright answers . . .

Preface: A Letter to You, the Family

Dear Friends:

My heart reaches out to you who have made, or are contemplating, one of life's roughest decisions—whether to place a parent in an institution. How well I understand your anxiety, your feelings of guilt, doubt, helplessness, and, yes, sometimes even resentment! You are not alone. At this very moment, thousands are struggling with these same emotions, emotions that can overshadow your conviction that "we're doing the right thing for Mother/Father."

I feel close to you because with my own parents, I, too, have known these feelings. After Father's stroke, my mother took care of him until this became physically too difficult. When he entered a nursing home, she was lonely, became disoriented, was glad to join him. But they were separated, placed on different floors, missed one another and the lifetime of living together. Father did well, continuing in his life role as a minister, helping with chapel services and with counseling. But Mother deteriorated rapidly, soon becoming bedridden.

I talk with you intimately about nursing homes not only as the daughter of parents who spent many years in an institution, but also from the vantage point of being a direct-care "nurse-who-nurses," that is, the licensed vocational nurse. Specializing in geriatrics and having worked in many nursing homes in many states as I trailed my mobile husband around, for years I have shared your joys and heartaches. With you I have rejoiced or agonized in every kind of situation—when my father fell out of bed, when my mother failed to recognize me, or when, for the first time in years, a nurse wheeled her outdoors to hear the song of a robin.

In observing nursing homes, my concern has increased for you, the relative, as well as for your parent, for, during these years, I came to realize that *your* feelings were seldom recognized; that your crucial role in the well-being of your parent was largely ignored, even though you were the connecting link with the outside world, to the memories and to a lifetime of give-and-take loving. Too often, without knowing why, you have felt helpless; you have not known what to expect or where you fit into the picture.

Now you will find out. Walk with me through the nursing-home door and discover many facts that you have a right to know—such as the "Six Common Practices," which may not be contributing to the overall benefit of nursing-home life and which hitherto have been kept in the realm of "professional prerogatives." Together we will tour that "nice" nursing facility up the street, to see whether it is just that, "nice," or whether it is a disaster. We will peek backstage both during and after visitors' hours, by day and in the dead of night, into every nook and cranny, to observe inner-sanctum events and attitudes. You will learn what to observe, and how to evaluate the care given. You will see how you, the family, can become a powerful influence in bettering that care. Our goal is high. For your parent, there must be total care of mind, body, and spirit. Nothing less will do.

Is it enough to know that the home is clean and attractively decorated? Is it enough that the staff seems friendly? You will see that these are merely basics to good care—that they are not enough when the total well-being of your parent is at stake. Most importantly, having defined your goals, you will stop wondering whether Dad or Mother lives a meaningful life or is simply existing. Gathering up new insights, you will find ways of coping with your wide range of feelings and how to put your sometimes misdirected, but marvelous, energy to constructive use.

Particularly in chapter 3, "A Mighty Fortress, the Family," the focus is on you—you who are the lifeline of your aging parent. May this period of your life bring satisfaction, growth, and a positive outlook for both you and your loved one. *Make your decision count.* Not only for your parent, but for *you.*

I am with you every step of the way.

Sincerely,

Nancy Fox

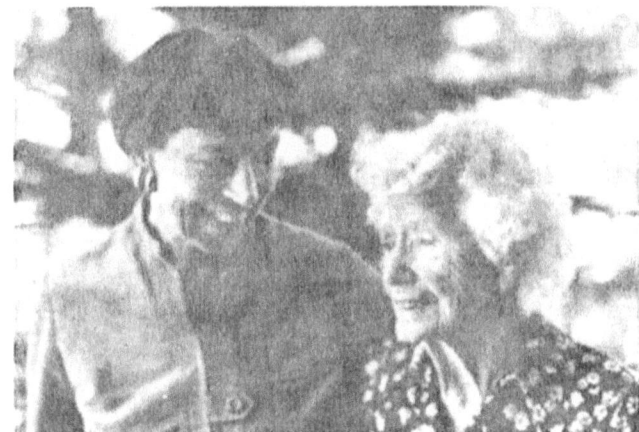

The difficulty in life is the choice.
George Moore

1
Filling Beds—or Filling Needs?

Thinking of a nursing home? Should you be? Are there other options for your parent? Keep in mind that institutionalization is costly, in both human and financial terms, and that if it can be avoided, it should be. But how?

Nobody knows better than you, her adult children, whether Mother* is suited to congregate living, whether she can adapt to institutional life. Of course, her own feelings are of paramount importance and will make the difference as to *if* and *how* she adjusts.

At this point, you and she are seesawing. To go or not to go to a home? From all sides, conflicting influences tug at you. You are wise—or you are cruel—to *think* of such a thing; she will love, or she will hate it there. From four sides you are bombarded:

---
*Mother or Father (or both). Women greatly outnumber men in long-term care facilities.

13

1) "Send her to a nursing home," says the doctor.
2) "You're just trying to duck your obligations," says the gossip.
3) "We have the bed for her—she'll love our homelike atmosphere," says the nursing-home industry.
4) "Consider *alternatives* to institutionalization," say citizen-action groups.

One-by-one, let us analyze these four points.

1) The doctor says that you should send her to a nursing home. Do you view this as a firm command that leaves you no option? Is this a carefully considered recommendation by a caring physician who is thoroughly acquainted, not only with your parent as a total person, but with the family circumstances? Is this order based on the best interests of the family as a whole? We trust that your parent is in the hands of such a conscientious doctor.

Or, could this recommendation be an "easy out" for a doctor disinterested in older people, who may benefit from lumping all his geriatric patients together? And consider, might this doctor even have a vested interest in the nursing home? "Doctors may own stock in nursing homes," says the American Medical Association, in response to my inquiry, "provided the patient has free choice of physician." The fact that doctors may own such stock, and that many of them do, is well documented, although some patients are in no position to make free choice of physician, especially those who have no family support.

Further, some physicians recommend nursing-home placement because they have neither the expertise nor the patience to arrange for or suggest alternatives for your parent. Witness the thousands of medically unwarranted admissions to nursing homes in the United States—up to 50 percent according to gerontologist Dr. James Peterson. Other researchers, such as Jane Lockwood Barney, of the University of Michigan, put the figure at 40 percent. And so, family, before blindly accepting the doctor's "send-her-to-a-nursing-home," make sure that first *you* diagnose the doctor; analyze his or her motives, ability to listen, to be concerned, and his or her degree of empathy for your particular situation. (Doctors will be further discussed in chapter 4.)

2) "You're shirking your responsibility to your parent"—the second influence—often comes as an over-the-fence rumor. There are always busybodies. As you weigh all the factors, you may find that the decision to enter your parent in a nursing home is a wise one. Unaware of the physical and psychological strain you are under, the gossips make you feel guilty, don't they! And you wish you wouldn't allow such people to derail you emotionally, knowing that such a decision would be harder on you than on your parent—that only as a last resort would you send her to a nursing home.

Family, ignore the busybody. Instead, join or organize a self-help group where you will receive support in facing the problems you encounter; where you can discuss openly your innermost concerns, hostilities, whatever, in a climate of mutual trust. Break up your isolation. By sharing, you may find the situation more manageable than you had thought; you will find new approaches, new doors opening to you. One such group, called CAPS (Children of Aging Parents), receives encouragement from the Los Angeles Division of the National Council of Jewish Women.

3) Next, the nursing home administrator says eagerly: "We have the bed for her. She'll love our homelike atmosphere!" For many nursing homes, "optimum occupancy" is the motto. Many have ready accommodations for, like June, the nursing home industry is "bustin' out all over." Colossal chain corporations, like weeds, are sprouting everywhere. Flat, low buildings like barracks or tall, stratospheric structures dot the landscape. Total expenditures for nursing-home care grew 148 percent between 1973 and 1979.* These expenditures, both public and

---

*This figure may be compared with an increase in the consumer price index of 64 percent and a growth in the gross national product of 81 percent (according to the Health Care Financing Administration, 1981).

private, soared from $500 million in 1960 to over $17 billion in 1977.

Says Michael LaConey, vice-president of Merrill Lynch Corporation and top analyst of health-care stocks, speaking on the TV program "Wall Street Week" (July 11, 1980), "The nursing-home industry is now even larger than the drug industry." He projects total expenditures for the industry in 1999 to be about $75 billion.

And so, hints the industry, send us your parent—in fact, send us your uncle, your aunt, your cousin, *anyone*—because our livelihood depends upon every bed being filled.

Consider yet another pull on your pocketbook and emotions—the industry's public-relations thrust. Viewing itself as God's gift to the Grand Generation, as benefactor to mankind (and for some, it *is* just that), the American Health Care Association* paints a rosy self-portrait. Harken to the average administrator's public-relations chant, implying that angels-of-mercy hover over each and every resident at all hours of the day and night; that residents "adore" our gracious, country-club atmosphere, our gourmet meals; and implying further that all, even the young, can and do live together in idyllic ecstacy, such as described in this AHCA brochure:

> Many people. Old. Young. Playing cards. Reading. Pursuing hobbies. Talking together. Laughing. Interacting. Given this situation and asked to name the location, you might answer: "A church activity, a family gathering, a community social." But you probably wouldn't suggest a nursing home. It's only natural. Historically, nursing homes have long been stereotyped as a place for the aged to go when there is no other place. Yet today's nursing home is for the young and old alike. It is for all convalescents—young and old—who expect to recover fully as well as for those who are in need of long-term care. The emphasis is on living. The aim is to help a person to care for himself to the

---
*Member facilities (about 75 percent of U.S. nursing homes) of the AHCA operate for profit.

best of his ability, and to return him to his home and community wherever possible.

And so, "come all ye faithful," the industry seems to say, "join our happy throng; blend with ours your voices in the triumph song."

Given the size of many institutions, how many can *really* be described as "one happy family"? And shouldn't we question the inference that many patients are returned to the community? "Once private funds are exhausted, and Medicaid assumes the financial burden, chances for return of a patient to his or her home are greatly diminished," says the General Accounting Office *Report to the Congress* (November 26, 1979)—particularly when rehabilitation efforts are not made on a regular basis. In the average geriatric facility, how much of the industry's self-promotion bears resemblance to the reality of everyday life in a nursing home? Yes, there is a bed for your parent. But fanfare from the nursing-home industry should not be a factor in swaying your decision.

4) On this fourth point—"consider alternatives to institutionalization"—you will find support from citizen-action groups and other organizations around the United States.* Find out about those community services that can either postpone or prevent institutionalization. In a moment you will read of possible services in your area, but first you should know about "gatekeeping" mechanisms that are taking hold around the country. Preadmission screening programs and methods of assessment of need vary widely. A General Accounting Office review identified two models. One prevents clients from entering institutions when community services are available, appropriate, and less expensive; this is done by denying public reimbursement for nursing-home care and by authorizing payment for appropriate community-based services. The second model discourages people from entering institutions by advocating community care wherever possible.

---

*See Appendix, page 169-175.

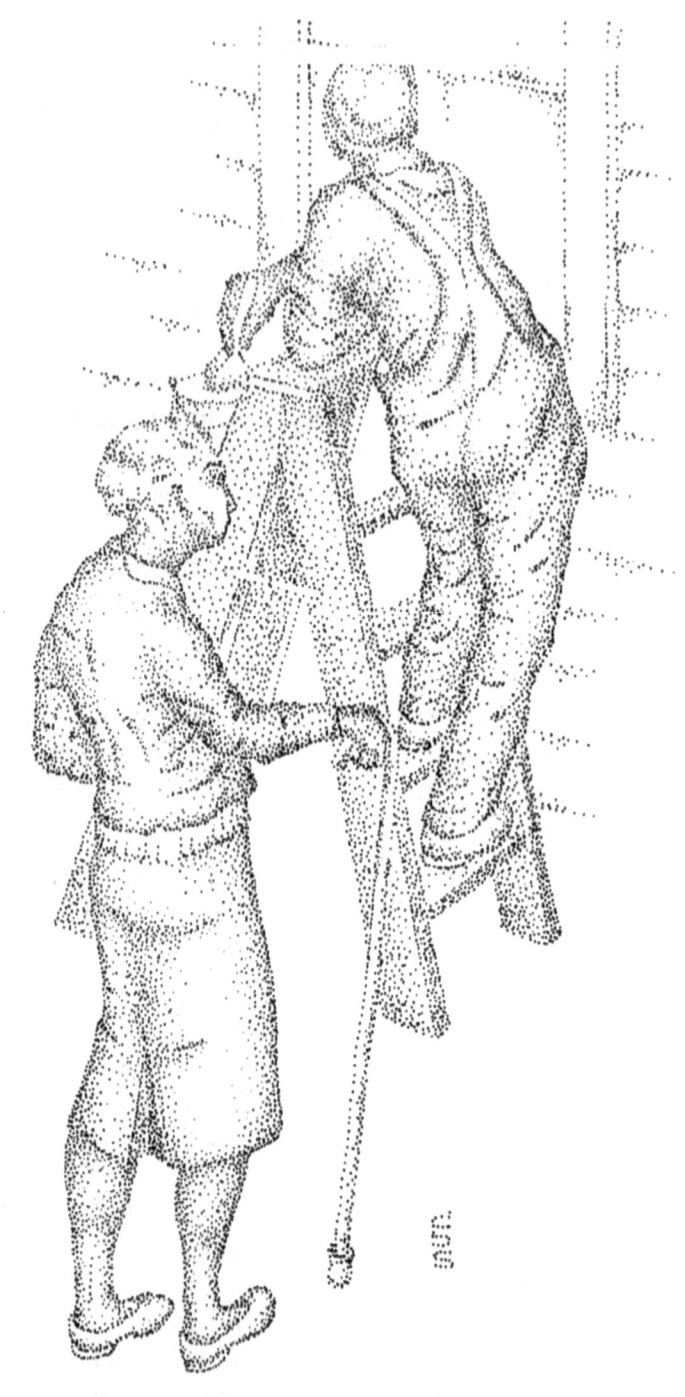

"We can't take complete care of ourselves so we live in a congregate home, doing what we feel we can do, receiving assistance in the tasks we cannot handle. We provide each other with company. We have our privacy and, within our limitations, we are independent."

The state of Virginia's preadmission program, for example, successfully diverted to the community 21 percent of its 3,592 applicants over a twenty-month period. The New York Monroe County ACCESS Project reported that 69 percent of assessed Medicaid clients and 58 percent of private-pay clients remained in the community.

Remember, the nursing home is a good idea for your parent only if all of the options listed below have been tried and exhausted, and only if family circumstances are such that home care or alternatives constitute too great a physical and emotional burden on the family. In short, for your parent, the nursing home must be a last resort.

Think of these community services as "stepping stones" that, used individually or in combination, can spare your parent the traumatic giant leap from home to an institution.

Community Services

home health care services
daycare centers
night sitters
grocery deliveries
volunteer visitors
dial-a-ride
meals-on-wheels
telephone reassurance
homemakers' services
live-in companion
handyman services
physician visits
visiting nurses
mental health counseling
home therapy
senior centers
family respite service
share-a-home
foster home

supervised apartment
retirement home
assistance from friends and neighbors
hospices

Having investigated the possibilities for these services through your local Information and Referral Service, listed in the telephone directory, or finding the appropriate services unavailable in your community, must you now consider a nursing home? Keep on looking, keep on asking questions. Contact your Area Agency on Aging—located in your state capital—or your local Council on Aging. We mentioned supervised apartments. In such a place, your parent can ring at any time for help, retaining independence; supervised apartments do not, however, offer nursing services. Or you may want to investigate the idea of low-cost housing, operated by HUD under the department of HEW (now called the Department of Health and Human Services).

Still another stepping stone would be the British "share-a-home" concept. In such places, four to ten older people share a large, renovated private home. Each resident has his or her own small "suite," and each shares in the total cost. The home is often managed by a warm, friendly woman who attends to meals and housekeeping. Here your parent can enjoy much of her own furniture and prized belongings, retain her independence, and continue to function in companionship with congenial people her own age. Responsibility for laundry and house cleaning is in capable hands. Here she resides in a more homelike setting than any institution could provide.

Visiting such a certified home in Trenton, New Jersey, I found a small group sitting outdoors in the lovely spring air, some crocheting to the music of a record-player set up near a window. The housekeeper, a buxom older woman, delighted in guiding me around the Victorian mansion, which she maintained in spotless condition. The aroma of bread baking in the oven filled the home. The song of a canary and a profusion of garden flowers, neatly arranged in vases, stirred the senses. Increasingly, the idea of "share-a-home" for older people is intriguing the American public.

On the list of community services, we mentioned family respite. What is respite care? An excellent example may be found at the Metropolitan Jewish Geriatric Center in Brooklyn, New York. Such programs are designed for older people who live in the community with relatives or friends who assist them in their daily activities. When, because of illness, vacation, or an unusual family situation, the family is temporarily unable to provide the necessary support, the older person can enter the geriatric center for a brief stay as a "visiting resident" until the family situation returns to normal. There may be such a service in your community.

Besides calling your Information and Referral Service, how else can one locate these community services? Which ones are available to you? The following agencies may be helpful in directing you to the various resources you wish to investigate:

    your local health department
    social security office
    senior center
    mental health association
    visiting nurse association
    Council on Aging
    Gray Panthers
    church and synagogue outreach ministries
    Red Cross
    family service agency
    Crisis Intervention Hot-Line
    daycare centers

Your Area Agency on Aging is listed in the Appendix. In addition, you might want to contact:

    Family Service Association of America,
    44 East 23rd Street, New York, NY 10010

    National Association of Home Health Agencies,
    426 C Street N.E., Washington, DC 20002

National Council for Homemaker Home Health Aid
  Services, Inc.,
67 Irving Place, New York, NY 10003

The American Association of Retired Persons,
1909 K Street, Washington, DC 20049

Gray Panthers,
3635 Chestnut Street, Philadelphia, PA 10104

Area Agency on Aging,
National Headquarters,
Suite 400, 1828 L Street, Washington, DC 20036

Having listed for you the many agencies available to assist you with the care of your parent, we must make it clear, however, that these services are not available to *everybody* who is in need of them. This dilemma is described by Bernard Sloan in the *Wall Street Journal* (July 23, 1981) as he related how his mother "made the mistake" of saving her money, disqualifying her from *any* form of government attention. He discovered that most of those marvelous programs were for somebody else and that, when he inquired about them, he was always asked: "Is she on Medicaid?" When he replied that she was not, government phones clicked in his ear. In a biting comment, Mr. Sloan observes that nursing homes in his area were filled with rich people who knew when to transfer their money so that Medicaid was footing their bills. And who was paying their costs? Those forced to supply their own care and do it all for themselves, "even while their hair was falling out, and they were throwing up, and their bodies were boiling with pain."

The Medicaid program, since President Reagan came into office, is facing curtailment, to the consternation of those patients who are not already excluded from its benefits. And again, as Bernard Sloan suggests, surely there must be a way to provide more basic help to people in genuine need, without penalizing those who have also worked hard, paid their taxes, and accumulated some reserves. To many persons, the question "Is she on Medicaid?" is like waving the red flag before a bull.

What, then, can you—the reader who is not on Medicaid—do about this? Write your congressperson. Send a copy of your letter to the American Association of Retired Persons (see Appendix, p. 169), to your Area Agency on Aging in your state capital, and to any group which addresses these kinds of problems.

Thinking of a nursing home? *Should* you be? Considering the alternatives you have investigated, the overall situation and condition of you and your family, as well as the state of mind, body, and spirit of your parent, how do you now feel about nursing-home placement? Will it fill your mother's need? Or will it merely be filling a bed?

Wise and prudent men . . . have long known that in a changing world worthy institutions can be conserved only by adjusting them to the changing times.

Franklin Delano Roosevelt

2
Sizing Up and Selecting a Nursing Home

You, your family, and your parent have carefully reviewed all aspects of your family situation. Now you conclude that nursing-home placement is the wise solution. Your next task? To find a good one, the right one for Mother; a home near enough so that, if at all possible, family ties can be maintained.

To help you make this choice, to compare, to find which type of home will best fulfill the needs of your parent, it is essential that you visit many facilities in your area. We divide them into four categories.

1) There's the "Villa Luxuria," a prestigious care home for those with a limitless pocketbook.
2) The "Geriatric Barracks," an oversized institution that operates on a rigid policy of routine and regimentation.
3) The "Geriatric Ghetto," a warehouse for the unwanted.
4) The "Home, Sweet Nursing Home," an individualized care home.

As you will discover, not all nursing homes fit snugly into

one of the above four categories. Characteristics may overlap. For example, you may find a "Villa Luxuria" that is highly regimented or a home that looks like a "Geriatric Ghetto" but that, in fact, provides loving care. Even a "Barracks" home, not *entirely* staffed by "top sergeants," may within its ranks include some warm, caring employees. Or, what seems to be a "Home, Sweet Home" may turn out to be deceptively cold and uncaring.

As you observe these places, extend your antennae beyond external impressions. Note what employees say and how they say it. Practice the art of hearing what is *not* being said. Note not only what is being done, but what is not being done. Picture your parent in each type of home as you consider the words of Jacques Guillaume: "Freedom to think and act as an individual is still one of the best ways to postpone incurable senility. Man is most likely to endure by becoming more and more individualized."

Our first visit is to the Villa Luxuria—one of the fancier facilities. Would your parent *want* to live here if cost were no barrier? Approaching such a residence, you walk through lush, too-green-to-be-true lawns, past the closely-clipped shrubs, and then ahead, through an arch of cypress trees, you glimpse the mansion. Arriving at the stately portal, you are greeted by a gracious hostess and escorted first through the lavish Louis XIV salon, then on to the ornate Oriental lounge—a feast of teakwood furniture, silk tapestries, rose medallion vases—splendor fit for an imperial invalid. Now you enter the high-vaulted dining room, Spanish in decor, to join a bejeweled dowager as she sips her fragrant Souchong tea. Next, you board a gilded elevator, and are whisked to an upper lobby, there to examine the residential suites where an aura of luxury prevails—costly carpets, oil paintings, chaises longues, potted palms. The nurses' stations are tucked discreetly behind an elaborate screen. Down the hall, young doctors stroll arm-in-arm with their aged "benefactors," chatting about golf, gardening—or perhaps Gauguin?

Extraordinary, too, are the therapy suites, another flight

up. Rehabilitation equipment, pools, exercisers—an apparatus of every description to coddle the body, for here, at the Villa, each client is socially and clinically worthy of a physician's time, a therapist's attention. In their autumn years, these residents seem remote from the slings and arrows of age which must be endured by many of their less fortunate contemporaries.

"Oh, to be old and affluent!" one might sigh. Here at the Villa a rather pleasant condition! And oh, the tender, loving care—all waiting for your parent, should she be admitted. Private nurses, doctors at her beck and call, saunas, massages, haute cuisine, *oui, Madame*—any luxury, just for her monthly autograph.

This is the Villa Luxuria, a nursing home of comfort and elegance. But, look deeper. Does it provide other than physical needs—more than just what money can buy? As you reflect on such questions, you will arrive at your own conclusions, but remember, whenever possible, include your parent in all decisions affecting her future.

Next, a visit to the Geriatric Barracks. A bed here would be more within reach of the average income. You see before you a group of long, low, flat-topped buildings, sprawled over a vast area. This institution, each unit cast from a common architectural mold, promises its hundreds of "enlistees" a regimen of routine, rules, and regulations. It prides itself on efficiency, on clockwork precision.

At the "barracks," modern technology is everywhere evident, especially in the loud-speaker system that all but eliminates personal contact between staff and patients. As a mammoth chrome food cart glides down the interminable corridor, you jump aside, watching with fascination as, automatically, it deposits dinner trays into each identical cubicle—machine-feeding each inmate.

Fantasy? Perhaps, but the assembly line of blank faces from which expressionless eyes gape tells you that in this facility individuality has been lost in mass treatment; that the "hup-two-three-four" approach to geriatric care, although easing management problems, has blanked out the human spirit.

Enough of the barracks, you say? That's not for Mother.

Your next visit uncovers yet another type of nursing home, the one that we call the Geriatric Ghetto. Entering the doorway, you cringe. It's a shocker. Despite government crackdowns, despite all the new legislation covering geriatric facilities, here is proof that the scandals exposed by the 1972 U.S. Senate hearings still exist today.*

Before your tour, the receptionist informs you that because of a recent change of ownership, this facility has been "greatly improved." At first glance, however, this is difficult to accept. What was it like before? Let me describe conditions in this so-called home as I found them several years ago in the city of Denver. Then we can compare.

At that time, part of my lasting impression was of dirty linens lying around, not only in the hallways, but in the main lounge. Stale and foul odors permeated the place. The gum-chewing staff, wearing dingy uniforms, were congregated at the nurses' station, where they laughed and talked—ignoring the moans of the old people who were wandering aimlessly around. On the tables, piles of dirty dishes were carelessly stacked, food dried on them. In a far corner, two half-naked men were lying on an unmopped floor. Feces were smeared on the wall of the elevator. With his feet propped upon his desk, the so-called activities director was leafing through a magazine.

Visiting the facility today, one would expect to find significant improvements, as promised. But no. Unpleasant odors still permeate the place. Residents still loll around, apparently overdrugged—with nothing to do or to think about. And again, we see the staff clustered around the nurses' station, socializing, oblivious to the loneliness and despair around them.

---

*Send for the latest free book from the Government Printing Office: #96-208, *Special Problems in Long-Term Care* (Hearings before the House of Representatives subcommittee on long-term care, October 17, 1979).

Some patients complain that they are not warm enough. I feel a few pairs of hands—ice-cold.

Improvements? Yes, there are some. Today, in the 1980s, the staff looks neat and clean. Beds are made, and no dirty linens lie about. Nursing care, whether provided or not, is adequately documented in charts. However, we still find old people not living, merely breathing. We continue to see minds and spirits as empty and forlorn as the outdoor chairs in winter; staff and residents alike are steeped in an atmosphere of despair.

But wait. You discover a bulletin board and read of stimulating activities scheduled for each morning and afternoon of the week. Perhaps you picked a wrong time to visit? You question members of the staff about that schedule. The conversation goes like this, typically, as you visit a Geriatric Ghetto:

"I see from the bulletin board that yesterday your residents went on a bus ride. Did they enjoy it?"

"Well, we planned to go, but the weather wasn't too good."

"Today you showed the Laurel and Hardy film. How many residents attended?"

"We were going to show it, but the film never arrived."

"I see that last Sunday you had church services, then took your residents for a picnic?"

"The clergyman never showed up, and the bus broke down."

"Well, you scheduled a bingo game for Saturday night. Did they enjoy it?"

"Nobody wanted to play."

If this so-called home has been "improved," we must wonder by whose standards. Even though there *are* signs of improvement, such as stricter criteria for cleanliness, we wonder whether we aren't still justified in labeling this a Geriatric Ghetto?

I believe we are. Impoverishment of minds and spirits still exists; staff apathy still prevails. Just as before, nurses and aides hold no belief in the potential, the capabilities, or the feelings of residents; they make no serious effort toward rehabilitation. Vacant eyes of patients bespeak lack of stimulation, lack of meaningful goals and pursuits, loss of incentive to live, shortage of staff. Residents merely exist. A frightening thought grips us. Are these "ghetto" residents any better off than a herd of cows put out to pasture?

On your next visit, you discover the Home, Sweet Nursing Home, possibly the kind of home in which your parent might thrive. This one, too, is far from perfect. Nursing homes are operated by fallible human beings, so no home will suit your parent in all respects. Still, we can call this one a "good" place to live, a "home" in the true sense of the word, where love abounds.

At first glance, you note that this one reflects the needs and tastes of its residents. Like the Marcus Garvey Home in Brooklyn, it abounds in living plants and flowers, tended by the residents themselves. With brilliant strokes of the pen, William Breger, the architect, has achieved a noninstitutional look such as is common in Sweden. You quickly discover what makes this place so warm, so inviting—the emphasis on sense appeal. Sensory stimuli are everywhere evident, linking pleasant surroundings to the well-being of the resident. Water fountains, goldfish, colorful artwork, percolating coffee, a pet cat in residence, the scent of hot rolls baking, the sound of music—all these living, moving, vibrant touches add to the aura of the home.

Something unusual that your mother will appreciate is the group of specialty rooms: one for residents who sew, with a cutting board permanently set up; others provide places to putter, write letters, and/or pursue hobbies. Here is a large, long table on which to spread out a stamp collection, make a scrapbook, spread out a map. Residents enjoy the quiet room, the large-print books, current magazines, and even toys for visiting children.* There are also a soundproof room for the

---

*In the Soviet Union, one nursing facility boasts a library of eight thousand books.

playing of musical instruments and a special room for baking, so that the residents, by providing refreshments for guests, may be givers as well as receivers.

In his book, *Body Language,* Julius Fast stresses the value of "space to call your own." Here at the "Home, Sweet Nursing Home," your parent would have "territory," that is, pride of ownership, the sense that she still has control over her own affairs, her own time, room for personal belongings that maintain her link with the past. Paradoxically, studies have shown that a private room encourages sociability. The resident can't wait to get out and mingle each day, whereas often, if a cubicle is shared (perhaps with a chronic cougher or uncongenial roommate), a person can lose a sense of identity and personal freedom. "Don't fence me in" is the silent plea. How does your parent feel about "space to call my own"? She should, if possible, be given her choice of a single or double room. It is significant here to note that in Norway, new nursing homes are required to have single bedrooms for 75 percent of their accommodations.

All nursing homes in our country either are operated for profit (proprietary) or are nonprofit (church, fraternal, or government sponsored). For a list of nursing homes in your area, write to your state department of health; to the American Health Care Association, 1200 Fifteenth Street, Washington, DC 20005, which represents the for-profit homes; or to the American Association of Homes for the Aging, 1050 Seventeenth Street, Washington, DC 20036, which represents the nonprofit homes.

In every state of the union, you will find both good and poor geriatric facilities, whether profit-making or nonprofit. And currently nearly 25 percent of the more than 1.3 million residents live in nonprofit homes.

Many of today's geriatric facilities have evolved from their historically negative image to the concept of "campus"—where clusters of buildings provide a wide range of services. The philosophy is to help people remain independent as long as possible. For example, the Philadelphia Geriatric Center consists of a hospital, two apartment buildings, a home for the aged, a research institute, and intermediate boarding facilities. They also provide a daycare center in another part of the city.

Other examples of the campus-type facility: the Carmelite Homes, Loretto Geriatric Center of Syracuse, New York; the Isabella Home Geriatric Center in New York; the Avery Convalescent Homes in Hartford, Connecticut; Golden Acres of Dallas, Texas; the Samarkand of Santa Barbara, California; the Lincoln Lutheran Home of Racine, Wisconsin; and Asbury Village of Gaithersburg, Maryland, to name just a few. One of the most complete and comprehensive nursing homes in the country, with an unusually wide variety of patient services, is the Byron Health Care Center in Fort Wayne, Indiana. Other homes, such as St. James Place, sponsored by St. James Episcopal Church in Baton Rouge, Louisiana, include private cottages, a clinic for minor surgery, and other services that allow for need and flexibility.

Years ago, as you middle-aged readers may recall, there was a place for the indigent elderly called the "poorhouse." My husband recalls when, as a child, he was scolded by his mother for foolishly spending all his allowance. She would point her finger at him and threaten, "Now Byron, dear, if you don't save your money, you will someday land in the poorhouse!" And little Byron would picture himself, aged eighty-five, in rags, crooked cane in hand, trudging up and over the hill into the sunset, forever consigned to the poorhouse, purgatory, and perdition!

Of course, the poorhouse was the forerunner of some of our old-age homes, now called "Homes for the Aging." As nonprofit organizations, they depend largely on voluntary contributions; and currently they have emerged, for the most part, as modern, progressive, service-oriented homes. Along with the for-profit homes, they offer a wide variety of services in accordance with the changing medical and psychiatric status of the older person.

How to Select the Right Nursing Home

- Obtain a catalogue of nursing homes from your state department of health.

- Shop well in advance for a home so that this is not a time-pressured, crisis-burdened choice.

- Visit a home without prior appointment. Ideally, make several such visits to a home that appeals to you, making your visits at different times of the day.

- The Freedom of Information Act has established the right of public access to nursing home inspection reports, on file in any district social security office. Take the time to check these out. For Medicare facilities, provider survey reports and statements are filed. Medicaid approved homes are listed at your county department of social services.

- In considering a particular home, ask the health department whether this home has ever received an "Intent to Deny License" because of uncorrected sanitary, fire, and/or patient care deficiencies.

- State licensure does not necessarily indicate adequate inspection systems. When was the last inspection made? By whom? With prior appointment? What qualifications did the inspectors have? Answers to such questions may be found through consumer advocate groups, through your state Ombudsperson, or through other concerned agencies listed in the Appendix.

Comparison Checklist

In choosing a nursing home, check several carefully and compare homes. (This compilation is in large part based on a government checklist.)

Name of Nursing Home A: _____

Name of Nursing Home B: _____

Name of Nursing Home C: _____

INITIAL QUESTIONS	A	B	C
Does the home have a current state license on display?			
Does the administrator have a current state license?			
Does the home have a history of serious violations from state reports? (Ask at social security or health departments.)			
Is the home certified to participate in financial assistance programs?			
Do current residents seem happy within the facility? Have they meaningful ways to occupy their time?			

(*NOTE: If the answer to any of the above questions is no, you should have serious doubts about the home.*)

LOCATION

	A	B	C
Is the home near a hospital?			
Is it convenient to family and friends?			
Is it convenient for the patient's physician?			

RESIDENTS

	A	B	C
Is a Patients' Bill of Rights posted in plain sight for all residents?			
Do residents have the right to speak and associate freely?			
Are they free to complain without retaliation?			
May they receive visitors?			
Are patients encouraged to vote in public elections?			
Do patients know where to make official complaints?			
Have they the right to worship freely?			
Are arrangements made for various religions?			

	A	B	C
Is there no discrimination on basis of race, creed, color, or national origin?			
Are patients used as test subjects only with their informed consent?			
Are physical restraints used only when ordered by a doctor—and is duration of use frequently reviewed by that doctor?			
Is the right to privacy respected? Curtain around bed? Is it used?			
Is there a telephone in a private location for patient use?			
Is there a place for private family visits? A privacy room?			
Are residents given reasonable freedom to decide "lights out" time—i.e., *not* "put to bed" at a child's early hour for staff convenience, then given sleeping pills?			

ADMINISTRATION

	A	B	C
Does the administrator know most patients by name?			
Is the administrator available to answer questions, hear complaints, or discuss problems?			

	A	B	C
Does the administrator spend most of his or her day at the facility?			
Are names and addresses of the owner and administrator available?			
Is the administrator courteous and helpful?			

NURSING SERVICES

	A	B	C
Is the facility adequately staffed day and night? Weekends? (See chapter 5, "Who Cares for Your Parent?")			
Is the staff turnover rate low? Have many on the staff been employed for over two years?			
Have adequate provisions been made for patient care during staff absence?			
Is a written patient-care policy kept current and available for each patient? Is it implemented?			
Are adequate records kept? (Check at your social security office.)			
Are thorough answers given to your questions?			

Sizing Up and Selecting a Nursing Home / 37

Is there a restorative nursing care program aimed at promoting independence? (See chapter 7, "Think Therapy.")			
Are RNs and/or LPNs (LVNs) on duty day and night? Seven days a week?			
Is there an isolation room for patients with contagious diseases?			
Do residents' visitors and volunteers speak favorably about the home?			
Are nursing aides paid more than the minimum wage required by the government?			
Is prompt care for the incontinent provided? At no extra cost? (Only the use of certain special equipment warrants any extra charges.)			

GENERAL PHYSICAL CONSIDERATIONS	A	B	C
Is the home clean and orderly?			
Is it free of unpleasant odors?			
Are rooms well ventilated and kept at a comfortable temperature?			
Is the general atmosphere warm, pleasant, cheerful?			

SAFETY

	A	B	C
Are wheelchair ramps provided wherever necessary, indoors as well as outside?			
Is the home free of hazards: obstacles to patients, unsteady chairs, underfoot hazards?			
Are there grab-bars in toilet and bathing facilities, handrails on both sides of hallways?			
Is an escape plan posted in a conspicuous place, showing all exits and traffic patterns, in case of fire? In case of other emergency?			
Are exit doors marked and easily opened from the inside?			
Are stairways enclosed and doors kept closed?			
Are fire extinguishers checked annually?			
Are hallways and ramps wide enough for two wheelchairs to pass easily?			
Are warning signs posted for unavoidable hazards, such as wet floors?			
Are rooms free of electrical cords?			

Are doorway thresholds flat?			
Are there call buttons within reach in rooms and baths?			
Is the home well lighted by day and night? Well enough for residents to read?			
Do beds have side-rails?			
Is the furniture sturdy?			
Are auxiliary lighting and power available for emergencies?			
Do bathtubs and showers have nonslip surfaces?			
Is there an automatic sprinkler system? Has it recently been checked?			
Are certain areas posted with NO SMOKING signs? Are these observed?			

MEDICAL SERVICES

	A	B	C
Are there adequate emergency procedures with doctor, ambulance, and necessary equipment available?			

Is there a medical director employed at the home?			
Are patients seen by physician at least every thirty days for the first three months and at regular intervals after that?			
Is there a public telephone within reach of wheelchair patients?			
Is the name and telephone number of the medical director furnished to patients and relatives?			
Are relatives notified prior to patient relocation? Is patient's consent obtained, wherever possible, before relocation? Relatives' consent?			
Does the home have an arrangement with outside specialized services, such as for dental, hearing, eye, and foot care?			
Is there a substitute always available for attending physician in emergency?			
Does the doctor actually visit with the resident, answer questions, and give emotional support during visits?			
Are pharmaceutical services supervised by a qualified pharmacist?			

FOOD SERVICE

	A	B	C
Is licensed dietitian on the premises often enough to adequately supervise planning and preparation of meals? (Ask to see the kitchen area in order to observe order and cleanliness.)			
Are meals varied, nutritious, appetizing, and served at appropriate temperatures?			
Are menus posted, and do meals conform to those menus?			
Are special diets available?			
Are religious dietary laws accommodated?			
Are meals served at appropriate intervals?			
Is plenty of time allowed for each meal?			
Are adequate utensils provided?			
Is prompt assistance given with eating when needed—at no extra cost?			
Is the dining room attractive and comfortable? Are there numerous small tables, rather than unsociable long ones?			

REHABILITATION ACTIVITIES   A   B   C

Question	A	B	C
Are evening as well as daytime activities scheduled?			
Are activities carried out as posted? Are field trips available? Are many residents given the opportunity to participate?			
Is there a large room available for special activities? (Check how often many residents take part in activities.)			
Are there group as well as individual activities?			
Are residents encouraged to participate—but not pushed?			
Is there a qualified recreational staff?			

THERAPY   A   B   C

Question	A	B	C
Is there a fulltime program of physical therapy available? Does a large percentage of residents take part?			
Are occupational and speech therapy, as well as names of therapists, available for all who need them?			
Are social services available to aid patients and their families?			

	A	B	C
Are mental-health services available for all who need them?			
Is there a varied program of recreational, cultural, and intellectual activities?			
Are activities offered for those who are relatively inactive or confined to their beds?			
Are barbers, beauticians, and masseurs/masseuses available?			

FINANCES	A	B	C
Is a written statement provided which details what is and what is not included in the daily rate?			
Is an itemized bill provided each month?			
Will the administrator give an estimated total monthly cost for an individual patient?			
Are there services which require extra charges?			
Are payment plans available and explained?			
Is a deposit required?			
Does the home have an adequate financial base?			

Is bonding provided for patient money?			
Are there adequate safeguards for patient's money and valuables? (Actually, it is best to take these home—watches, rings, etc.)			
Is there an adequate policy to compensate for personal possessions lost or stolen?			
Does the home concur that relatives need to bring an attorney when signing contracts?			

OTHER AREAS OF THE HOME	A	B	C
Does the home have an outdoor area where residents can get fresh air and sunshine? Is it often used?			
Is there a lounge where patients can read, chat, play games, watch TV, or just relax—away from their rooms?			
Are visiting hours convenient for patients and visitors?			

Unto whomsoever much is given, of him shall much be required.
The Gospel according to St. Luke 12:48

3
A Mighty Fortress, the Family

In olden days, family ties were rock-solid. A mighty fortress was the family unit. If you asked a Jewish child his name, he would first give you the name of the family settlement or village where he lived, then the family or tribe name. Finally, if you persisted, he would tell you his given name. It might sound like this: Nazareth Horowitz Isaac. Back then, the generations were linked. Members stayed, played, and prayed together. And for grandmother, the nursing home was a concept beyond her wildest imaginings.

Today, families are likely to be scattered, mobile, strangers to one another. Divorces are common. To their grandchildren, today's elderly may be unknown. And when a birth, funeral, or anniversary occurs, a partial family reunion may take place once a year—or once every ten years. "Who are you?" says one cousin to another, "and what do you do, where do you live?"

Fortunate is the aging person of today who, upon admission to a nursing facility, feels that he or she has the support of a close-knit family—one who sticks by him, visits faithfully, remains vigilant to his concerns, and vocalizes reactions to the nursing-home staff when pleased or displeased by the care being given. A mighty fortress . . . *your* family?

Visit, be vigilant, vocalize—the ingredients for inner peace, both for your parent and for your family. We will elaborate shortly on that threefold formula; but first, does the following scenario strike a familiar chord?

Today you took Mother to the Hilltop Convalescent Center. Yes, you feel awful. As you kissed her goodby—oh, that forlorn look in her eyes! How she clung to you! And now, flopped on the sofa, you relive that painful parting. Suddenly you cry out: "John, what have we done—thrown Mama to the wolves?"

A lump blocks your throat. Mother is so precious, but oh, the way she'd forget to turn off the oven, or watch for cars; the way she would trip on the step. And that eternal reminiscing! But Mother was so special—did I say "was"?—so brave about her leg pain, so loving with the great-grandchildren. And her parting words—"Ellen, why must you put me away?"—they haunt you.

Torn by the mental seesawing, "Oh, Mama," you groan, "as a child when I was difficult, you never put *me* out to pasture!"

The dam breaks. Pressing your face against your husband's shoulder, you sob your heart out and then, exhausted, fall into a troubled sleep.

The next morning, things look brighter. After all, you realize, Mama hasn't flown to Mars. Once she is oriented, she will be fine. But, of course, you feel guilty! Everyone does, at first. Guilt, however, is a luxury you can't afford. Don't forget that while Mother was at home, you did your very best by her, given all your other family and community responsibilities. It wasn't easy—of course, you sometimes "blew your stack"; but face it, couldn't she, at times, try the patience of a pope? Show me a family without blowups and I'll show you hidden hostility. The point is, you were close, you were loving. Nothing has changed. Mother is still very much a part of the family, that is, *if you will let her be.*

Let her still be part of the family? But how? First, shed that guilt. Put your pent-up energy to good use. Plan for Mother a meaningful future. How?

Here is your formula. Latch on to the three "V's"—watchwords for any family of an institutionalized person:

- visiting
- vigilance
- vocalizing

Let's consider these in more detail, one by one.

First — visiting. As you are not a "dump-and-run" family, visit regularly. To give Mother the joy of anticipation, let her know when you are coming. And you teenagers, never forget that Grandmother is special — she is your roots. From now on it is your job to keep the generations linked. Have you heard of Charles Percy's Volunteer Youth Corps? Each week, young people like you bring in to the nursing home a piece of the outside world — sharing games and snacks, reading aloud, writing letters, running errands, and such. The delighted residents dress up, perk up, and eagerly await the coming of "our dear young people." Listen to what your elders have to say. Encourage them to talk, to tell you about the historic old days they knew so well. They can teach you much about life.

When you visit as a family, be sure to take the little ones — the great-grandchildren. I knew a mother who refused to expose her children to "all those crippled people" — a good way to cripple the attitudes of her own young ones! Instead, teach them early that to love is to reach out. Children find beauty in a face, no matter how timeworn. Residents long to cuddle a child on their laps. Your parent wants to remain part of the family.

How might you prepare a child for a visit? Adapt these Easter Seal Society suggestions to the child's level of understanding:

1) Remember, the nursing-home resident is a person like anyone else. He or she has only the special limitations of his handicap.
2) Give help only when requested.
3) Let the resident set his or her own pace in walking and talking.
4) Avoid stopping and staring. He or she deserves the same courtesy as anyone else.
5) Avoid being overprotective. No pity or charity.
6) Try not to ask embarrassing questions. Take care not to separate the nursing-home resident from a needed wheelchair or crutches.

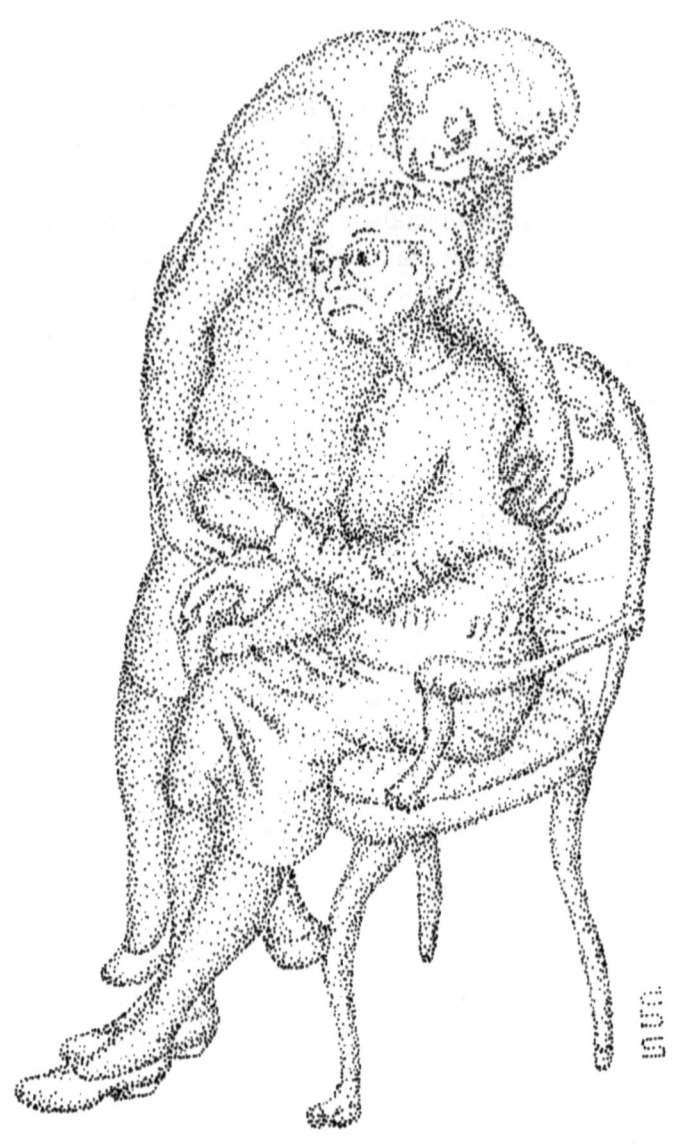

"These are my quiet years. I can't run bases as well as I once could, but I want you to understand that I can still give you the wisdom of my experience."

7) Enjoy your friendship with the handicapped. Their philosophy and good humor will give you inspiration.

The second "V"—vigilance. Tune in to all that happens in the nursing home. It *is* your business. You are not an "outsider." She is your mother, isn't she? Relatives have a right to a ringside seat in all that affects a parent's well-being. Be vigilant! Monitor the care she receives. Use these guidelines:

The doctor: How often will the physician check your mother? Keep track of the number and length of these calls. And since these calls are important and costly, make sure her doctor is conscientious—not one of those hello-goodbye-doorsill doctors. From the head nurse, obtain regular reports on her condition. Do not hesitate to call the doctor when you need further explanation.

Medical orders: What drugs, if any, are prescribed for your parent? Exactly what for, and for how long? Are these prescriptions for the less costly, but just as effective, generic names, rather than brand names? Get a list of all obtainable generic-name drugs from your pharmacist.

Nutrition: What diet is ordered? Is this precisely what your parent is receiving? Are posted menus identical to the meals served? Unless contraindicated, what about bulk in your mother's diet? Does she get roughage, or just soft, squishy, constipating foods which necessitate laxatives?

Are real fruit juices served instead of sugary imitations? Crisp, fresh salads? Green, not overcooked vegetables? Whole-grain breads? Milk? Decaffeinated coffee? Does she eat alone or in company with others?

Exercise: What has the doctor ordered? Why or why not? As inactivity promotes sluggishness of mind and body, does she get this exercise as often as prescribed? Wheelchair patients, too, should get regular exercise.

Recreation: To sustain her joy of living, is Mother included in recreational, spiritual, and cultural activities? She'd rather not? Forcing, of course, is out; but ask whether and how, in the first place, the opportunity was offered. Is therapy a part of her care plan? Why not? Again we remind you, this is a convalescent home, not a boarding house, not a hotel. What are the goals of her therapy plan? Is occupational therapy just busy-busy work, or is it meaningful to her—such as making something for deprived children or pursuing an already-established hobby?

Roommate: Has Mother a congenial roommate? Good. This is essential. No? The situation must not persist. This kind of daily stress demoralizes one and inhibits rehabilitation. (I know of two women who always sat back-to-back, never conversing. You could cut the hostility in the air with a knife!)

Mother's room: Does the home allow personal furniture, pictures, treasures? If this is a "home-away-from-home," she needs these vital links to her past. These help her to retain her individuality.

We have seen from these ideas how your parent may feel that, far from being "put away," she remains part of the family. In giving up Mother to the nursing home, you have not given up on *her*.

Your third "V"—vocalizing. Speak out whenever Mother has a legitimate complaint. Silence sends out false messages. Let's say Mother is agitated because she keeps getting cold, slimy eggs for breakfast. Will she herself complain? No, according to a Scottish survey, most residents feel that the staff is too busy, or they hate to rock the boat. And so, the job falls on you. You will find that the staff does better by the patient whose family shows it cares. A good home welcomes your concern, *wants* to set things straight.

Or, let's say you are hearing that "short-of-help" excuse too often. Rather than fume because Mother is not receiving the care you expect, make an appointment to see the head nurse. Talk it out. If you do not receive satisfaction, go to the administrator. Do not become intimidated if the blame is put upon "finances." Your parent is paying for health care, that's why she is here—that's why the nursing home is called a "Health Care Center." Patients' rights include the right to services for payment rendered. (But remember, services can also mean that the staff tries to enable your parent to do as much *for herself* as possible—to let her retain independence.)

Whatever you do, talk it out in a friendly manner. Cooperation? It is far better to cooperate than to have to take your grievance to outside sources.*

To cushion complaints, an Oregon facility sponsors a Family Forum—a monthly gripe session attended by staff, families, and all residents able to attend. Doctors and administrators are urged to come. Through honest dialogue, minds are stretched, viewpoints aired, frustrations dissolved. Cookies and lemonade lighten the atmosphere. Patients find that as individuals, they do count; staff keeps open channels of communication; families feel that they are playing a vital part in the life of the home. The Family Forum is an idea which is taking hold in many facilities across the nation. Does your parent's facility provide such a forum? For the resident who has no family, a volunteer or "backup" fills the gap, as described in chapter 10, "For Your Parent, Life More Abundant."

In vocalizing, convey your gratitude, too, for what you like about this home and its hard-working staff, many of whom are dedicated. Show your appreciation for the loving atmosphere. Do the aides exhibit unusual sensitivity to patients' needs? Tell them so. Surprise the head nurse, the activities director, the dietitian, housekeeper, or doctor with a "good-for-you" letter. And they will see you as an ally, concerned that this home be not just a dreary dead-end, but a life-affirming place where each resident looks forward to tomorrow.

Others have felt the same guilt. Here is the way one relative expressed it:

Apologia:**

To the Nursing Home Staff from the Children of Your Patients

Know that we truly love those we commit to your care—
   the loved ones we've tried so hard to provide for.
If we sometimes act indifferently it is only to hide our aching hearts.

---

*See page 153.
**From *The Journal of Practical Nursing*, Vol. 30, p. 32, February 1980.

Try to understand our grief, our sadness, our guilt, yes,
   even our shame, when we are forced to face our limitations
   and turn to strangers in our helplessness.

We have struggled long and hard and it is not easy for us
   to surrender our bittersweet burdens
   to those we do not know.

Try to understand our torment—we hate ourselves for doing what
   we must do as much as our parents hate us
   for abandoning them in a strange place.

Forgive the anger of our agony when we lash out at you
   with our petty grievances and unreasonable demands.
   It is the circumstances of our being here that we resent—not you.

We do not mean to burden you with our needs
   but sometimes our frustrations overwhelm us.
   Perceive, if you can, our hurt and please be gentle with us.

We appreciate all you do for our parents—the love and
   care and kindness you show them.
   We envy your being able to do for them what we no longer can do.

And when we fail to express our appreciation
   it is not because we are ungrateful,
   but because by so doing we are forced to acknowledge
   our own uselessness to our parents.

Are you still wondering whether your mother will receive good care to dignify her remaining months or years? I promise you this: Much depends upon you, her family—her "mighty fortress," her bulwark never failing. If you use your powers of observation; if you become her watchdog, guided by the messages of the forthcoming chapters, yes, for sure, Mother will receive the best of care. And you will find new freedom and peace of mind which, at this period of your life, you richly deserve.*

---

*If, because of distance or other reasons, you cannot provide the supports we have discussed in this chapter, whom can you delegate as your backup to assume this responsibility?

Let no one suppose that the words **doctor** *and* **patient** *can disguise the fact that they are* **employee** *and* **employer**.

George Bernard Shaw

4
How to Diagnose the Doctor

> This chapter is dedicated to those physicians who show concern for the elderly *no less* than for other age groups.
>
> It focuses, however, on the premise that the time has come for the medical profession, as a whole, to look more carefully to the medical and psychological needs of the institutionalized elderly.

Having stressed the importance of physical surroundings, we will now talk of the psychological environment of the nursing-home resident. The relationship of staff to the well-being of patients is well documented in the literature, for, as you realize, staff attitudes can promote either joy or gloom, indeed can influence a patient's will to live.

We begin by getting to know your parent's physician. A crucial question: How does this professional feel about attending a geriatric patient? To what extent does he or she feel concern when giving orders for diet, exercise, medication, rest, and therapy? When making life or death decisions? Learn about this doctor and his attitudes. Does he hold rigid, universalized concepts of aging that negate the quality of the individual, consigning the patient to a useless generality? Does he harbor low expectations of the older person that may rub off on the staff, affecting *their* behavior toward their clients?

Or, is he a life-affirming physician, one who grasps the rehabilitation potential of your mother and who respects her as a person—characteristics you have a right to expect in a doctor—why else is this professional associated with the field of geriatrics?

As a lay person, you see the need to diagnose the doctor. To do this, you will receive guidelines as this chapter progresses.

First, it is necessary to understand that the relationship between your mother and the *family* doctor may or may not be ongoing, once your parent is admitted to the nursing home. In some geriatric facilities, at your specific request, it may be possible to retain your family physician. Otherwise, she will be under the supervision of a doctor on the staff of the home. Before admittance, be sure that you and your mother understand clearly the provisions for medical services.

If you are involved with a Medicare-Medicaid certified institution, the doctor is required to visit every thirty days for the skilled-care patient, every sixty days for the intermediate-care patient.

Be on hand, when possible, when the doctor visits your mother. At other times, discuss your concerns with the RN in charge. If you cannot arrange a time with the doctor, write him a note, expressing any specific questions you may have. Include your telephone number and address and ask him to call you for a conference.

You may have heard a doctor say, "Now, John (or Millie), what can you expect? It's your age!" The rationale that a patient is too old to benefit from therapy, surgery, or rehabilitation measures may be a clue to a doctor's inability to grasp the vast potential of creative geriatric medicine.

Our hope is that your parent will be supervised by a competent, approachable physician, one who is knowledgeable in the special field of geriatric medicine, one who reflects his belief that a person is never too old to be comfortable. (We have seen an 89-year-old in a dentist's chair, receiving a new set of "lowers.") Quite frankly, many a doctor takes no interest in the older patient.

Check the credentials of the medical staff by using these references at your local library: (1) *American Medical Dictionary,* an alphabetical and geographical index; (2) *Directory of Medical Specialists,* a directory of physicians certified by the Boards of Medical Specialties; and (3) *Biographical Directory of the American Psychiatric Association.*

Although since January, 1978, nursing facilities have been required by law to provide a medical director, we need not remind you that *caring cannot be legislated.* Learn about this professional, who can swing in any direction your parent's wellbeing. Remember, too, that the physician is handsomely remunerated for services rendered and, as sometimes happens, for services merely charted but *not* rendered.

Gazing into the mirror, a doctor can be hypnotized by what he or she sees—a "haloed healer," high on a pedestal, who claims to provide (although in many areas, statistics disprove this) the best health care in the world. But do *all* patients see this rosy reflection? Some see no image at all as, on them, the doctor pulls his vanishing act. You have heard the frustrated pleas of many an aged person: "But *where* is my doctor—why is he always unavailable?" Is there anything harder than the softness of indifference?

In an article published in the journal *Prism* (voice of the American Medical Association), one doctor admits to this "plain indifference." U.S. Senate investigators, however, put it more bluntly in their report. "Abandonment" they called it. That was nearly a decade ago. Today, the dilemma for the older generation still exists to a frightening degree. That report—"Doctors in Nursing Homes: The Shunned Responsibility"*—

---

*See "Special Problems in Long-Term Care" (Appendix, page 169).

should serve as a warning to you, the family, to maintain your vigilance and to "know thy physician."

To alert you to certain practices among some professionals and to spare you, not only money, but various degrees of heartache, let me document some actual case histories. Fortunately, because of staff vigilance, not all of these patients were losers in the lopsided battle of the healer versus the helpless.

Case One: The Doorsill Doctor

Mr. Groves, aged 88, was in severe pain. Strange black markings appeared on his chest. Nurses repeatedly called for the doctor. Days later, when the doctor finally came, he did not enter the patient's room but merely stood at the doorsill and questioned the nurse. He ordered an arthritis medication. Days passed. A son, infuriated by the lack of medical attention, demanded that his father be hospitalized. X-rays revealed three broken ribs.

Case Two: The Stunned Nun

Sister Marie, 78, became dizzy and bewildered. Her eyes wandered. She would lunge forward, her head flopping into the supper tray. The doctor ordered her to be restrained with a safety belt. Sister Marie was humiliated.

Even more humiliating to the nun was her increasing loss of bladder control. She was scolded by aides (an approach most head nurses would not have condoned). The patient was sufficiently aware of the situation to be highly embarrassed.

The fact was, Sister was overdrugged. Her medication orders were never challenged. For months, the doctor remained "unavailable." Shrugged the aides: "My, but Sister is getting more senile every day!"

Finally the doctor appeared. It was only then, at the suggestion of a newly-employed Geriatric Nurse Practitioner

(GNP), that the medications were discontinued. Sister reverted to her normal, alert, articulate self. The restraint was removed.

Case Three: "Just Keep Him Comfortable."

Branding Mr. James as "hopeless," with "nothing more you can do," the doctor charted as follows: "Aged. Senile. Incontinent. Nonambulatory. No treatments recommended. Prognosis poor."

That was seven years ago. Today, Mr. James, aged 91, is alive, well, bright-eyed, in control of bodily functions. He walks without assistance, sings, smiles, reads, enjoys TV as well as occupational and physical therapy.

Somebody disregarded the doctor's evaluation. Somebody cared enough to initiate rehabilitation, inspiring the entire staff to participate. Somebody refused to cheat Mr. James out of his right to good care that would elevate him to his highest capabilities and potential.

Case Four: A Fact of Age?

When I questioned the premature death of Mrs. Littell, aged 78, her doctor rationalized: "Among other reasons, she was covered with infected bedsores."

Then a lay person, accepting the physician's word as law and viewing bedsores as "a fact of age," it never dawned on me to check her skin. Today, with nurse's training and realizing my rights as a relative, I know better. Bedsores? In this enlightened era? *There is no excuse for bedsores.* They are painful, preventable; yet, as confirmed by a government report, they flourish in countless nursing homes staffed with skilled people. And because Mrs. Littell was maintained in a drugged stupor, she could not complain. She remained most of the day in bed—without exercise. Rapid deterioration was inevitable.

I knew this patient well. She was my mother.

Case Five: The Ping-Pong Patient

Mr. Samson, 79, suffered not only a foot infection, but an unavailable physician. After fruitless efforts to summon the doctor, I phoned the clinic and explained the problem. I informed them that I had put this man in a taxi, accompanied by an aide, and that he was on his way to the clinic for treatment.

One hour later, Mr. Samson returned. No treatment. No medical orders. Returning him to the clinic, this time I pled more urgently for examination of his foot. Our staff feared gangrene. But again, forlorn as ever, Mr. Samson reappeared at our doorstep.

By now I was livid. With no intention of making a ping-pong ball of this man, I returned him to the clinic—this time insisting, "He is to have *immediate* emergency attention!"

At that, a new voice took over the phone: "Who in hell are *you*, and by what right do *you* order *us* around?" It was Doctor Martin. "Never mind who I am," I retorted, "just you treat Mr. Samson or I'll report you to the city's highest medical authority! Plus I'll have a report on this in tomorrow's newspaper!"

Two hours later Mr. Samson returned to us. Judging from the impressive foot bandage he sported, we deduced that he had indeed received tender, loving care. The aide handed us a note, indicating treatments and medications prescribed. And our Mr. Samson, beaming all over, handed me a slip showing the date and time of his next appointment.

Case Six: "She Belongs in a Nuthouse!"

Like wildfire, this under-the-breath proclamation by a midwestern doctor spread through the long-term care unit. He meant Mrs. Snyder, who was receiving verbal and physical insults from the ancillary staff, and who, with all the vigor she could muster, retaliated with punches, biting, and kicking. On my first day of employment as floor supervisor, the sole briefing I received from the head nurse was: "Be careful of Mrs. Snyder.

She belongs in the nuthouse!" As commonly happens, the doctor's attitude had rubbed off on most of the staff. And I wondered: "Does your remark mean, Doctor, that Mrs. Snyder actually should be transferred to a state hospital? If not, have you any notion as to how your attitude toward Mrs. Snyder has influenced the staff in their treatment of her?"

Despite all, this tale ends happily. Somebody cared enough to "bother" with this person, to draw out her long-dormant traits of gentleness, humor, self-esteem. Once again, this woman learned to smile, to draw us into her circle of love as we drew her into ours. She belonged, it seems, not in the "nuthouse," but back again with the human race.

It is a pity that the one person who can significantly upgrade the quality of patient care in a nursing facility and simultaneously improve the morale of both patients and staff often absents himself from the scene. That individual is the physician. This is a major problem with U.S. nursing homes. The U.S. Senate Subcommittee on Aging puts it this way: "The need for physicians to exercise greater responsibility for the over one million patients in nursing homes is abundantly clear...."

Case Seven: Buried Alive

In another facility, Mrs. Sorenson was buried alive. Or so it seemed. Paralyzed, frustrated by loss of speech, for two years she had been isolated in her room. Insensitive to her feelings, the staff assumed that she could not hear, see, or think. At times, when this woman needed urgent medical attention and a nurse would dial for the doctor, the staff snickered: "The doctor? You're kidding! When he comes to see *her*, that'll be the day!"

One afternoon I asked an aide to wheel her outdoors. Being

newly employed, I was dismayed by the girl's reaction. "Not me," she cried, "what would people think!"

Wheeling her out myself, I made a discovery. Mrs. Sorenson *could* speak—that is, with her eyes. Deeply expressive, they conveyed enchantment as she watched the flutter of a butterfly, inhaled the scent of a lilac. However, upon our return to the unit, her serenity was shattered. Out of nowhere came a voice: "Old Sophie there—she won't last much longer!"

Mrs. Sorenson's face flushed. Her eyes, darting right and left, sought assurance. Rushing her to her room, I held her in my arms—but it was too late.

Two weeks later the doctor did come, but only to make the pronouncement. For this time, Mrs. Sorenson was not alive.

Case Eight: "No-Nonsense Nora"

Sitting in the clinic, Nora Smith was on time for her appointment. However, she had to wait. She waited and she waited. For two hours past the scheduled time she waited. Finally, irate, she stomped out the door. Back at the nursing home she wrote this note to her doctor:

> Dear Dr. Weldon,
>
> I, too, was once a professional person. Now, as then, my time is valuable—as precious to me as yours is to you. That will be $40.00 for my wait in your clinic. My charge is $20.00 an hour. Please remit promptly.
>
> Sincerely,
> Nora Smith, Sunset Home, Room 59

Conceding this round to "No-Nonsense Nora," the doctor remitted—and promptly.

As these cases and much other sworn documentation

reveal, shortchanging the geriatric client is not uncommon among physicians. Some reasons:

Foremost is the fact that negative societal attitudes toward the retired and aging permeate every stratum of our culture. Doctors are part of this society. They, too, hold fast to many myths concerning this stage of life, such as, "You can't teach an old dog new tricks."

Secondly, it is well known that the curriculum of U.S. medical schools largely neglects geriatrics and gerontology. (Gerontology, as you may know, is the study of aging in all its aspects.) At a time when the aging population is escalating rapidly, this foot-dragging is inexcusable. Of the 132 U.S. medical schools, very few *require* geriatrics or gerontology as part of the curriculum. (The state of Ohio takes the lead in this respect, with a legislative mandate that each of its seven medical schools must incorporate geriatrics in medical training.) Approximately two-thirds of U.S. schools offer geriatrics, but only as an elective subject. Almost one-third fail to offer this training at all.

Dr. Robert Butler, president of the National Institute on Aging, is concerned about this foot-dragging. He proposes the creation of "teaching nursing homes" as counterparts of "teaching hospitals," to help the nation gear its research and training capacities to the needs of the growing elderly population. He calls for a public-and-private-sector partnership to develop teaching nursing homes in cooperation with universities, saying that this would do much to counteract the general view of geriatrics as the medical/nursing "pits"; of aged clients as "crocks"; and of old age as a "hopeless, useless time of life."

We see, then, that the negative attitudes of our society plus the lack of physician education contribute to the nursing-home problem. To the average medical student, geriatrics holds no glamour, offers no dramatic cures, rarely makes the headlines. Remuneration, especially in rural areas, may be considerably less than what he or she would like—nonetheless these are the areas where the geriatritian is urgently needed. For example, in McCook, Nebraska, a recent count showed only five doctors for ten thousand residents, whereas in Bend, Oregon, in the beautiful Cascade mountain area, there were eighty-two doctors for twenty thousand residents.

Those doctors who *are* interested, but who merely apply the physiological approach, are helping their clients do no more than "walk backwards into the future."

To the imaginative student, however, geriatric medicine (which encompasses prevention, rehabilitation, and its own unique approach to drug and other therapies) can be a challenging, creative career, highly rewarding in personal satisfaction. So let us now look on the brighter side. To stimulate interest in geriatrics among students who train in their hospitals, the Veterans' Administration has established a geriatric fellowship program in twelve VA medical centers around the United States. In addition, it is exciting to see the many gerontology centers springing up over the past decade at many of our universities. But this is just a starter. We need to go a long way in these directions.

To arouse people's awareness, public TV's program "Over Easy" strives to develop more positive attitudes and understanding of the aging process and its challenges. And Hugh Down's book, *Thirty Dirty Lies About Old* (see Appendix, page 169), can be enjoyed by all members, young and old, of your family. Again, on the positive side, a segment of the "Today Show" (NBC, October 16, 1981) told of a group of doctors in New York who provide what they call "gericare," or low-cost care to the elderly. After the Medicare payments are made, they charge so little to patients who come into their clinic that the older people are delighted and surprised. (Dr. Jonathan Kagan, ophthalmologist, was narrator.)

Although for some physicians geriatrics offers little incentive, these same professionals somehow elicit from their clients a doctor-worship cult. A classic example of the doctor-worshiper was my elderly friend, husband of one of my patients. Although complaining bitterly to me, when his wife died, that neither he nor she had set eyes on the doctor in five months, this man posted a paid notice in a local paper, saying: "I wish to thank

Dr. Vale for all his kindness and excellent care of my wife." Confronting him head-on, "For goodness' sake, Jack," I asked, "in view of your complaints, why the card of thanks in the paper?" "Oh," came the sheepish reply, "here in the midwest, that's the customary thing to do."

To the nursing-home patient, the doctor is a pillar to lean upon—a star in his or her sky—not just for physical ailments but for emotional support. When a resident is slighted, or thinks he is, the hurt is real and contributes to low self-esteem. It would be prudent, then, for you and your family to have an initial understanding with the physician so that expectations are kept on a realistic level. You will need to know the frequency, length, and day of those regular, legally-required visits. If there is delay or postponement, ask that you be informed in advance. (I have seen patients cry out in anguish as time and again their hopes for a doctor's visits were dashed.)

Will Mother get her money's worth or will she be stuffed into one of those "gang-visits," that is, dozens of superficial checkups within one hour's time, after which the doctor tosses out medical orders as glibly as one scatters seed to the birds? (One such whirlwind doctor met the plea of a dying patient with the advice, "Aw, Carl, all you need is an outing with a glamorous blonde!") Until more physicians accept greater responsibility for the care of long-term clients, stories of negligence will continue to be told.

We now laud those physicians who are faithful to their long-lived patients; doctors who understand that unless there is healing of hurtful emotions, there can rarely be comfort or cure for the body. All honor to the doctor who, forgetting to gaze into the mirror, finds it only natural to enfold within his or her professional circle those who, as Pearl Buck described them, "have come a little farther in the experience of life."

All honor to the doctor who, although he may not be religiously inclined, helps the elderly draw strength from religious belief. In his book, *Respectful Treatment: The Human Side of Medical Care*,* Dr. Martin Lipp asks a patient in stress,

---

*Hagerstown, MD: Harper and Row, 1977.

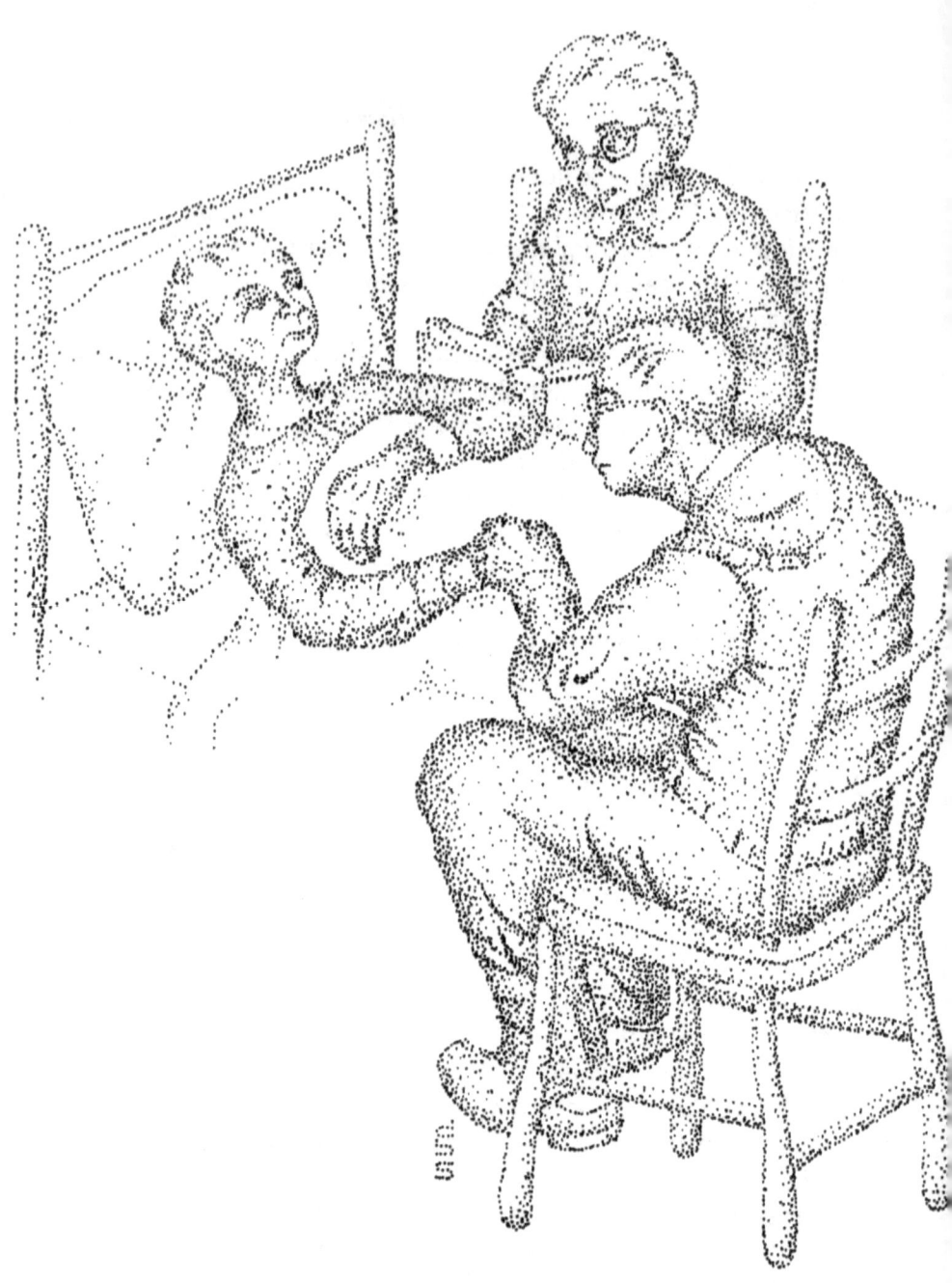

"We have started a reading group and together we read and discuss the old loved books and the new ones. Lately we've expanded our range and we read at the bedside of some who can't join our circle."

"Have you ever found comfort in prayer?" If to this patient this has been helpful in the past, the doctor then asks how he would feel about saying a prayer now, even asks him to pray for all who work on the health care team. Without exception, this has resulted in greater calmness and a closer therapeutic relationship between doctor and client.

Can a physician give good care without respect for the patient? Continues Dr. Lipp: "If you don't respect the process of giving care, how can you respect yourself? Disrespect for the patient may be ultimately more harmful to the doctor than to the client. I need to value what I do," he says, "even if the patients don't think they need it for themselves."

A good physician will stress the importance of these measures for your institutionalized parent:

- Eye care (Glasses fit? Regularly checked?)
- Ear care (Hearing aid used? Properly maintained?)
- Foot care (The right shoes? Special care for diabetics?)
- Skin care (Bedsores? Itching? Dryness?)
- Dental care (Properly fitted dentures?)
- Balanced diet
- Mental-health counseling, if necessary
- Exercise, encouraged daily
- Therapy or rehabilitation (Enough of each?)

Residents have the same right to these services as do any other persons in our society. Inability to pay should not deter the availability of such services. The health-care facility is not a hotel. It exists in order to furnish *all* the health-care needs of its residents.

You have met and diagnosed the doctor. Feel free to ask questions, to be informed as to the exact status of your parent, and to monitor her care. Another caution: Beware the haphazard diagnosis that, even today, some physicians cannot seem to shake off—that is, the use of that wastebasket term *senile*. This is a word that fails to represent a medical conclusion drawn from careful examination of your parent's nine body systems plus findings of laboratory reports. If there is a sign of mental confusion, find out what is known about it, what is being done, and how you can assist your parent in her therapy.*

We wish you—the family—satisfaction in your relationship with the doctor . . . that geriatrician who cares (with genuine concern, let us hope) for your mother.

---

*See chapter 6, "Is This Senility Necessary?"

All work is empty, save where there is love.
The Prophet

5
Who Cares for Your Parent?

Who cares for Mother? Let it not be a staff who thinks of residents in terms of "dealing with" them, "tolerating" them, "handling" or "putting up with" them. Let it not be staff members who shrug, "You either like them or you don't!"

Let those who care for older human beings be those who understand the sanctity of life—those who, through their special training, sensitivity, and ability, *make meaningful* the lives of those we call the "Grand Generation." Let it be those whose reverence for human life calls for health-care services in the context of physical, psychosocial, and spiritual dimensions. Each aspect of care, as they know, enhances the others.

Who cares for your parent? Let it be a staff that works well together, that stays, plays, and prays together . . . a staff sensitive to the unspoken needs of their clients . . . a staff who feel especially called to this challenge. Finally, let it be those who not only *care for*, but *care about*, your parent.

1) The Nurse-aide (or Nursing Assistant)

We first spotlight the nurse-aide, who takes direct care of your parent. (Nurse-aides account for nearly 89 percent of the nursing care staff—although this ratio is changing in some facilities which are using more trained and professional nurses.) Often overworked, underpaid, and often unacclaimed, just who are these aides and orderlies who work in American geriatric facilities? How important is their work? How qualified are they to care for other human beings on a daily basis? Observe their behavior. Would you want one of them to take care of *you?*

Qualified? The nurse-aide *must* be qualified, for that person wields a powerful weapon—the power of kindness over abuse, hope over despair, dignity over degradation, joy over gloom. The aide brandishes a sword that can strike life or death to the human spirit.

Does the facility properly screen and train these persons on whom it pins so great a responsibility? Does it not only require comprehensive, continuing in-service training, but demand pre-employment classes for all new applicants? The law has requirements, but are they enforced? Some facilities require only two weeks of instruction before salaries start. Others require more, and still others permit the new employee to go directly on stage without first learning the lines, although most states have now banned this practice.

When you consider the skills (listed on pages 77-78) needed by a nurse-aide, how much emphasis do you think should be placed on pre-employment training?

We speak here not merely of training for helping with the physical care of your parent. Some homes settle for far too little in the realm of psychosocial approaches, failing to utilize community-sponsored workshops and pre-employment courses offered. To put the "rookie" right to work without sufficient previous exposure to geriatrics and gerontology is not in the best interest of the client, even though that nurse-aide may be under supervision most of the time.

The new aide may bring to her job misinformation about aging and the elderly. She may subscribe to societal myths—to what Dr. Robert Butler, president of the National Institute on Aging, refers to as "ageism," meaning prejudice or discriminatory attitudes toward the elderly. These attitudes will very likely be communicated to the residents. Further, due to lack of adequate training, many in-home accidents as well as many insults to the patients occur. These accidents and insults are caused by the inexperienced, immature personnel who, in many cases, have never before set foot in a long-term care facility.

Why is pre-employment training downplayed by certain facilities? An example of this reluctance toward adequate education comes from Florida where, although in 1979 dozens of programs to train aides were funded in the state's vocational and technical training schools, most nursing-home operators were not utilizing the offerings. As a consequence, the Chairman of the House Committee on Health and Rehabilitation Services had to demand that the nursing-home industry meet with members of the Department of Education and the State Ombudsman Committee to develop recommendations for aide training through these schools.

In many areas of the country, pre-employment courses are offered by community colleges. Or, as in Minnesota, to augment in-service training, the Gray Panthers conduct a series of seminars for nursing-home personnel. Topics include ageism, sexism, racism, assertiveness, effective communication techniques, and the positive and negative uses of power. For information on the availability of pre-hiring training for nurse-aides, call your Department of Health or Social Services. This matter of training is an area of top concern for patient-advocate groups, who have seen how deficiencies can cause trauma—even to the extent of episodes of horror such as happened in a small midwestern geriatric home—as follows:

Tammy, without previous training, was scheduled for solo night duty (the nursing home was seriously short of staff and two staff members had called in sick). The girl was instructed to phone the charge nurse should problems arise. Alone with forty patients, the girl was frightened. Making rounds at 3:00 a.m., she entered Mr. Morton's room to find him panicky, struggling for breath. Aghast, his roommate looked on. Moments later the breathing ceased. The man fell back, lifeless.

Emitting a howl, Tammy fled to the nurses' station, too dazed to dial for help. There she sat until the arrival of the 7:00 a.m. shift. Still crying, she bolted, never to return—not even to collect her paycheck.

How can such episodes occur? They can and do, which brings us to that "short-of-help" syndrome that afflicts countless institutions. Accustomed to the excuse "We're short of help," shouldn't you, the relative, examine its implications? Translation: Short of help means simply this—*short of care*. It means that accidents can happen in so-called care homes. It means that people fall out of beds, chairs. They break bones. Fires flare up. Patients wander away and get lost. Trays are removed before clients finish their meal—sometimes even before they touch their food. People fall downstairs when a staff member is too rushed to lock the cellar door. People are killed in accidents in the "health care" home that is short of staff.

Not enough supervisory staff? Beware the administrator who intimidates the complaining relative with: "Well, now, if you don't like it here, you can always take your parent somewhere else."

Short-of-help has other implications. Nurses and aides are short of time. They stagger under a workload that is impossible to complete. This results in short tempers and a high turnover rate that can average more than 75 percent a year. And what about staff rights, such as the freedom from pressure on the job, freedom from having to work a double shift, or parts thereof? Such pressure on the staff obviously affects the residents, is unfair to clients who have the right to quality care for payments rendered. Can such a home accurately be called a *care* home?

In many ways, the good home, adequately staffed, serves the public well. However, to fulfill its promises, *every* home must attract and retain sufficient staffing on all three shifts, weekends included. This must and can be done. There is no excuse. "But," you ask, "how much is 'sufficient'?" Here is how you can tell if a home is short of staff:

Look around at the residents. Are they lolling all day in beds? Many dressed only in robes? Sitting hour after hour, in wheelchairs doing nothing? Parked mindlessly before a TV set; placed along corridors, back to back, grabbing at anyone who passes by, just for attention? Again, you know the home is short of staff when you search all over and cannot find a nurse or aide. This may happen especially on weekends.

To confront this shortage, here is a first step. The idea of a locked-in minimum wage for nurse-aides must be abolished. Hiring practices must be upgraded to curb turnover, to provide training that teaches not only physical care, but how to put joy, creativity, vitality into geriatric practice, and how to enhance the psychological well-being of each resident. Minimum wage? What does this tell you? What does it tell the nurse-aide? Simply that his or her work is not worth much; that she, as a person, is not worth much; that the residents who have reached old age are not worth much. Looking at it this way, is it any wonder, then, that low self-esteem runs rampant among ancillary workers? Low self-respect can lead, and all too often does lead, to patient abuse, whether verbal or physical.

The wise administrator and board of directors, then, will abolish using the minimum wage as set salary and will set up a promotional ladder so that the nurse-aide has goals to which she can aspire, something that increasingly is being done in some states where the charge-aide is especially trained and the Geriatric Nurse Practitioner is employed. Generally, however, aide work is a dead-end job without sufficient fringe benefits. The only escape? The employee quits.

Some nurse-aides quit because of family or child-care problems. We know of a highly successful approach to this problem, taken in the Milwaukee, Wisconsin, area, where a day-care center is provided for children, right on the nursing-home grounds. Employees have no worry about their children and the nursing home residents are visited each day by the tiny tots, to the great joy of all concerned. Staff turnover has been cut to a minimum.

Many nurse-aides can be called "jewels." Meet one such person, Nelda. Loving, imaginative, here is a conscientious worker. I recall the sizzling afternoon when the air-conditioning system collapsed. Patients were sweltering. Nelda requested a twenty-minute leave from the premises. Noting the gleam in her eye, I agreed. Upon her return, she wheeled the chair-bound residents into the lounge, put on the record, "I'm Dreaming of a White Christmas," and then . . . glancing up from my desk, I had to chuckle. For there they all sat, purring like cats, each licking a scrumptuous chocolate ice-cream cone!

And I remember Joan. Volunteering back- and footrubs, lending an ear to the lonely and troubled, she helped them to know the comfort—

> . . . the inexpressible comfort
> Of feeling safe with a person,
> Having neither to weigh thoughts,
> Nor measure words—but pouring them
> All right out—just as they are—
> Chaff and grain together—
> Certain that a faithful hand will
> Take and sift them—
> Keep what is worth keeping—
> And, with the breath of kindness,
> Blow the rest away.*

Creatively working to promote greater independence in her clients, Joan is an inspiration. She reminds us that "the purpose of all help is to make help superfluous."

Among nurse-aides, you will find Neldas and Joans, but also, some like Hilda, who are unmotivated, plodding along in low gear, losing every chance for personal growth. I remember

---

*Dinah Maria Craik, "Friendship," *Best Loved Poems of the American People* (Garden City, NY: Doubleday & Co., 1936).

the day when, balking like a mule, Hilda refused to join the sign-language class. Unlike her colleagues, she will never know the joy of communication with old Mr. Todd, who, stone deaf, is isolated in a world of his own. Then, alas, you may encounter Beulah, the Block-Aide. She's the one who blocks innovative measures and concepts in geriatric care. "We've always done it this way," she insists, "and that's good enough for me." Ignoring the needs of heart, mind, and spirit, she continues to believe in "*Body care*—that's all I'm hired to do."

Hickory-dickory dock, this aide watches the clock. The clock strikes three (or seven or eleven) and pfft! Like a cat at the sound of "scat!" she scampers out the door, too rushed to grant Mrs. Carr's request for a glass of water. Already halfway down the street, "Let the next shift get it," she hisses.

On the other hand, happily, many nursing aides who are caring and conscientious deserve credit. You will marvel at the stamina of those whose inner drive impels them, year after year, to continue on the job. We commend them. The work is exhausting.

Another point about hiring practices in nursing homes: There is a crucial need for orderlies, not only to do the heavy lifting and transferral of residents from bed to tub to chair and the like, but to give personal care to male clients. Would not a helpless man (it could be your father) prefer to be bathed by another male? Many an older man, stripped of his clothes by an immature young female aide, feels stripped, as well, of his dignity. He either submits or violently objects to such assistance. And yet, most homes fail to attract orderlies. A decent wage could make the difference. Here, again, citizen-action groups are protesting, for, as clearly stated in the Patients' Bill of Rights (see page 150), the patient's dignity must be preserved. Male patients, so embarrassed over receiving help from an aide who herself probably despises the assignment, beg to have their baths cancelled. And, similarly, orderlies complain when assigned to assist female patients for baths, showers, dressing, or undressing.

Poor hiring practices contribute to the high turnover rate. New faces constantly appear on the staff. How is it where your mother resides? A high turnover rate of staff bodes ill for the home's reputation. And although some staff members remain faithfully on the job, continuous orientation of new personnel not only wastes their time and administrative money* but affects continuity of care; and a vicious circle develops—using only minimum wage, which leads to staff turnover, which leads to clients bewildered by the ever-changing faces of their caretakers. You might well hear a patient wail: "But who will take care of me tomorrow?"

Laxity in hiring practices? Perhaps it starts with the way a facility advertises for help. Check the classified ad of your local paper. Does it say: "Aide wanted for the 'X' nursing home"? Hardly inspiring! This type of ad is likely to attract the "ambling Annies" who, with rundown heels, saunter into the office smacking a wad of bubblegum. "If you can't get a job anywhere else," Annie giggles, "you can always get one in a nursing home." Hired on the spot and often without references or training, within a month she may quit or be fired. But since many homes are short of help, they may keep her on, regardless of competence. Perhaps, however, the home runs a different kind of ad: "Seeking just the right person for Nursing Assistant. If you are gentle, willing to learn, respect the elderly, we need you." I have seen that ad in Christian Science publications. This time it is a well-groomed Susan who applies. Thoroughly screened as to her motivation, qualifications, and references, when selected, Susan takes a pre-employment geriatric-aide course sponsored by her local college or health department. She grows in her profession through constructive, ongoing in-service education, taught by an enthusiastic, demanding nurse. Susan regards the upgrading of her skills not as a "drag," as one aide described it, but as an exciting step toward mastering the art of

---

*Turnover cost for a Wyoming long-term care facility from January to June, 1981, was $18,000.

not just physical but "total" care. Relating well to residents and staff, holding her head high, she is proud to tell you, "I am a Nursing Assistant."

A government study found that nursing homes should be more selective as to whom they hire. What happens when "help" is hired off the streets? I will not spare you the following episode, taken from my own experience in an eastern nursing home.

Mr. Garcia had just expired. An aide and orderly, both high-school dropouts hired without references, were assigned to prepare the body for removal. Passing by his room, I paused to say adieu to this brave, kindly old man who had met his death with serenity. I was unprepared for what followed. The aide was giggling over the antics of the orderly who, to exhibit his manliness, ballooned his biceps, yanked out the in-dwelling tubes from Mr. Garcia's body, lifted the body upwards and outwards so that it landed with a thud on the stretcher, the impact causing the head to bounce. Three times it bounced off the pillow. Hooting with glee, the two young people then grabbed the cart, pushed it out the door, their raucous voices diminishing in volume as they disappeared down the hall.

When greater care is shown in the screening and selection of applicants for the position of nurse-aide, when paychecks reflect their ability and experience, we may expect greater interest; we may see the more serious-minded person applying for the position; we may see people who will exhibit greater job satisfaction. The result? Fewer turnovers, and therefore better care, not only for the elderly but also for younger clients who may also be found recuperating in nursing homes. Only a special person can be a nurse-aide. Not everyone has the heart, mind, and strength.

Many nursing assistants are sensitive to the needs of their charges. We depend upon them. Your parent cannot manage without their help. Without their services, nursing homes would close.

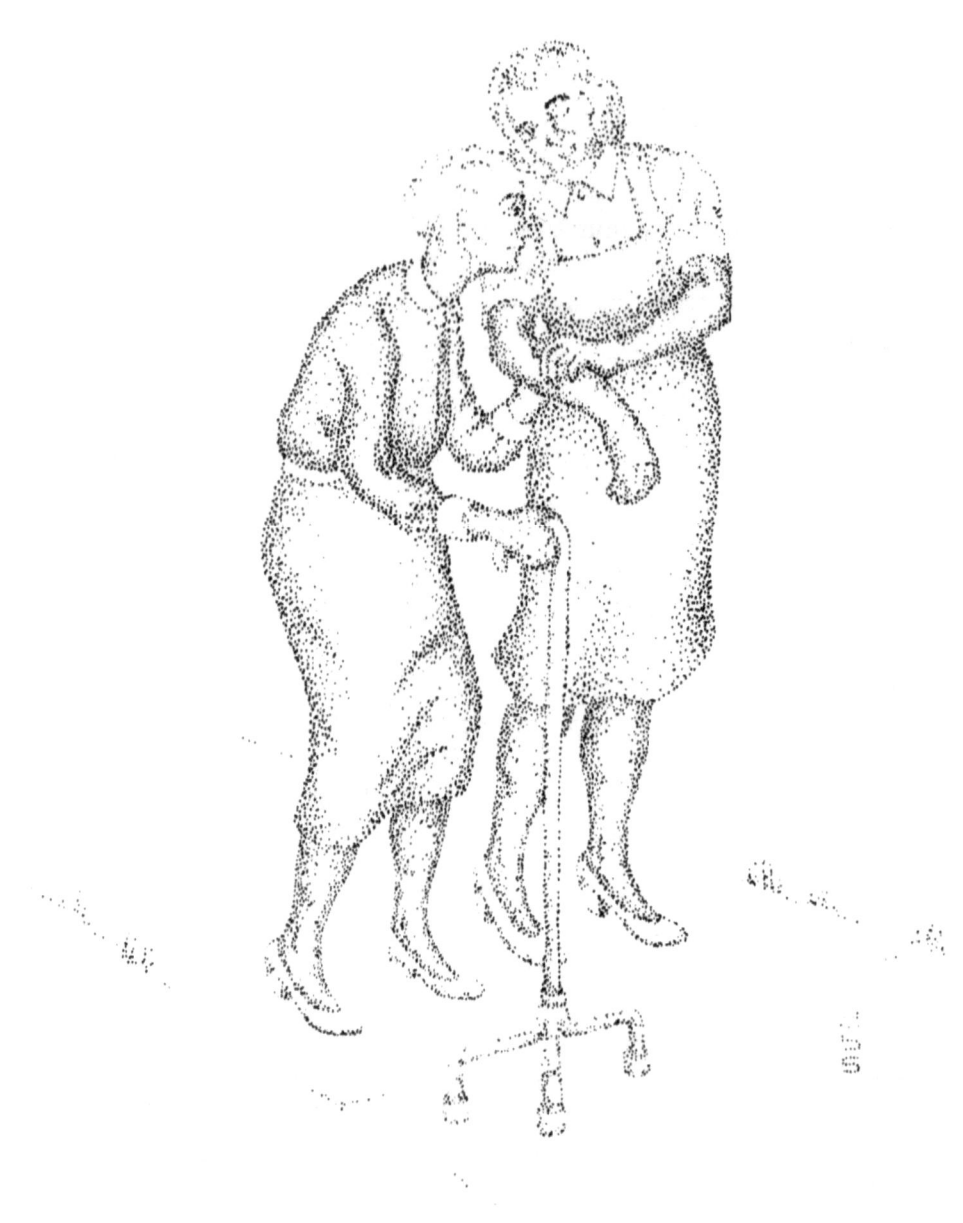

"My legs are not as strong as they once were so now I lean on your arm and when you're not here, I walk with a 'walker.' I do for myself as I am able and ask for assistance when I need it."

Specifically, nurse-aides must be thoroughly trained in the following essentials of long-term care:

- Understanding of the myths and stereotypes of aging
- Skills in nonverbal communication
- Understanding of problems caused by sensory loss
- Skills in maintaining continuous reality orientation for each resident
- Skills in listening and observing
- Ability to adjust one's pace to that of the resident
- Ability to spot and report signs of fatigue
- Ability to provide support in emotional crisis
- Ability to reawaken dormant interests and hobbies
- Ability to maintain the self-esteem of the incontinent resident
- Ability to encourage without nagging or anger
- Ability to see each resident as a unique individual
- Ability to respect complaints and anger and to deal with them honestly and constructively
- Ability to refer to a resident in a respectful, positive tone
- Understanding of sexuality, at any age, as part of being human
- Ability to speak directly *to* a resident, rather than *about* him, when in his presence
- Ability to spot any self-destructive tendencies in a patient (and awareness of the need to report these to the head nurse)
- Awareness of the need for good lighting
- Awareness of the need to maximize a resident's independence through self-help
- Awareness of a resident's possible need for spiritual counseling
- Awareness of the importance of privacy and modesty for each resident
- Awareness of the need for a happy, serene atmosphere
- Willingness to use first names—however, *only* with the consent of the resident

- Respect for the dignity of each resident
- Understanding of the special needs of the terminal patient as well as those of his or her family and roommate(s)

And, finally, let us briefly consider a model program for training the nurse-aide. You, the relative, may want to bring this program to the attention of the administrator in your parent's facility.

MODEL TRAINING PROGRAM FOR GERIATRIC AIDES

Inadequate training of personnel explains in large part why the nursing-home industry fails to provide the level of care expected by the American public. One successful training program is found in the Kansas City Gray Panthers' Geriatric Aide Program, 2937 Lockridge Street, Kansas City, Missouri 64128.

Creator, organizer, and director of the Kansas City program, with an advisory board of twenty-two members, Mrs. Mildred Barnes herself had once received only a sketchy orientation in preparation for a job as aide. The course she planned calls for two hundred hours of classroom work plus clinical experience at a local nursing home. It introduces the student to the physiological, psychological, and sociological aspects of the aging process and of attitudes toward the elderly. Special emphasis is placed on patients' rights.

A broad base of community support was developed through the advisory board, representatives of community, church, and health organizations, as well as senior citizens and other consumers. We consider this an excellent model program because of its strong emphasis on the psychosocial care of the nursing-home resident. Although primarily designed to promote an understanding of physical skills, it reaches far beyond that to higher levels of understanding—the intellectual and spiritual needs of the elderly person—in order that he or she may not only exist but live each day in a meaningful, creative manner.

Which nurse-aides care for your parent? Let them be the Neldas and the Joans, those who uphold the sanctity of life, provide tender, loving care; those who through their unique training and talents freely give of themselves to enrich the autumn years of your parent.

Who else cares for your parent?

2) The Nurse

"What kinds of nurses supervise my parent?" you wonder, as you picture the "angel-of-mercy," immaculate, gentle, soft-spoken—that caring lady-in-white. But wait! This picture implies outdated assumptions.

Lady? Not necessarily. In the 1980s you will find the male geriatric nurse very much with us. He, too, can inspire devotion and motivation, and can provide excellent nursing care.

In white? Again, not necessarily. "This is a 'home,' not a hospital," say some administrators, who see the white uniform as sending out a subtle "think-sick" message. Your parent may see a staff attired in pastels—any hue of the rainbow.

Angel-of-mercy? Well, you hope so. Most nurses are like that. But remember Nurse Ratched, in *One Flew Over the Cuckoo's Nest?* Kind, yes, *if you don't question her authority;* sympathetic, perhaps, *except for a touch of sadism;* a veritable Florence Nightingale, possibly, *but don't suggest a change of routine, or venom spews from her mouth.*

It is difficult to judge a nurse before your parent is under her care. What if you encounter a Ratched? Or one who may simply be inconsiderate? Or less than competent? Need you accept this? In chapter 3, "A Mighty Fortress, the Family," you have already considered what you can do when a nurse's attitude affects the well-being of your mother.

On the other hand, you may encounter Miss Rae—perhaps a Registered or a Licensed Practical/Vocational Nurse. Surely you would want *her* to care for your mother for, like ginger ale, she sparkles, puts joy and creativity, not mindless routine, into her work. She loves older people and shows it. With open eyes and ears (she seems to have at least six of each) she observes your parent—her likes and dislikes, hobbies, past interests, her whole family. Miss Rae also takes note of your parent's church affiliation or synagogue, her former lifestyle, her travel, and other experiences. You like the way this nurse makes you feel welcome, day or night. Miss Rae is the charge nurse, and, as she goes, so goes her staff. In fact, so go the physicians who visit here.

If the "gang-visit" doctor cuts short a visit to any one of Miss Rae's patients, he or she would encounter the wrath of this head nurse. Like a lioness, she guards her cubs. Woe unto the doctor who invades her territory simply to diagnose a client as "senile," douse him with drugs, then disappear.

"Doctor," Miss Rae insists, "why no rehabilitation orders for Mrs. X?" Or she will say, "Why has Mr. Y been on 'that drug' since the Year One?" Miss Rae has even been heard to complain, "Tell me, Doctor, why the tranquilizer as panacea for every geriatric problem from deafness to dandruff, hoarseness to hangnails?" And although this nurse works in cooperation with physicians, Miss Rae does not hesitate to remind them that this is the age of the geriatric nurse's lib. Indeed, it is nurses of her caliber who have helped to bring this about.

Today's emphasis is on gerontology and geriatrics, on new research, on literature that upholds the older person as an individual with greater potential and mental capacity than we had believed. Increasingly the families of clients can be less apprehensive about placing a loved one in a nursing home. Over the past few years there is evidence that societal attitudes toward the aged are changing, as well as attitudes of health-care employees. Hear what one nurse, Marion Boward, says about these changes as she relates her struggle to bring about new approaches. (Printed with permission, the following letter was first published in *The American Nurse* magazine.)

Dear Editor:

... here's one nurse, for nine years in a 132-bed facility ... the dilemma I experienced is probably representative of most of us who had the courage to enter and the fortitude to stay in the arena when a nursing-home position was very low on the scale of preferred preferences.

It was often a day-to-day dilemma of challenging the administration on accepted patient-care practices—or—of not rocking the boat by overlooking inadequacies. ... It was the dilemma of whether or not to acquiesce to forces firmly dedicated to the status quo. It was the dilemma of slipping quietly off to another job or keeping faith with the voiceless.

And that was the strongest bond. ... I stayed. And now, my voice has been joined by many others. A new administration heralded the opening of many doors. Because I struggled so long with so many diverse problems, I found myself catapulted into a central leadership position. Nursing administration is now the chief patient advocate and functions as the inter-disciplinary head in planning and implementing patient care. We had nowhere to go but up, and our coattails are flapping in the breeze.

We, as a facility dedicated to the staff-patient-community concept of responsibility, are on the move.

If I sound enthusiastic, I am! Here I stand, looking into a future which makes the past seem worth it all.

        Sincerely,
        Marion Boward, R.N.
        Director of Nursing Services
        Homewood Retirement Centers
        Williamsport, Maryland

Marion's story of hope and revolution has been repeated in

many American nursing facilities. May your parent be blessed under the care of a nurse who sees the resident not as a faceless number, deserving only custodial care. (This is the dangerous notion that she needs only to be fed and kept safe, which results in both physical and mental impairment.) Instead, may the nurse in charge of your parent take the high road, finding joy in making her comfortable, stressing her abilities rather than her disabilities, preventing further complications. May this nurse identify your mother's potential for rehabilitation, enhance her dignity, include her in planning, allow her participation in her own care, give her choices—for example, "Would you like your nap now or later?"

In short, may she have nurses (Registered or Licensed Practical/Vocational) who uphold her life at a significant level of meaning. Rest secure if you entrust your parent to a Nurse Marion or a Nurse Rae.

Today, through national nursing organizations, the nursing profession strives to sharpen its goals, to define and redefine its standards of practice—a sign of vitality within the profession. The Licensed Practical Nurse (or, as he or she is called in western states, the Licensed Vocational Nurse), because of her direct involvement with bedside care, is known as "the nurse who nurses." And today she trains for many responsibilities that only a few years ago were the exclusive prerogatives of the Registered Nurse. Together, as indispensable members of the health-care team, both LPNs and RNs help to meet the health needs of the nation. How do you evaluate the nurses who care for your mother?

Increasingly, nurses such as Marion Boward are placing great value on geriatric care as their professional preference and commitment. The 1970s welcomed the advent of the Geriatric Nurse Practitioner, or GNP, as he or she is called. While trained for traditional nursing knowledge and skills, she has acquired additional skills for which she is certified—such as interviewing, physical assessment, diagnosis, and treatment of common health problems of the elderly. Recognizing that the nursing of older people varies from that required for younger groups, and understanding as we do today that geriatric care must encompass the holistic (mind, body, spirit) approach, rather than just the physical, the health-care team gladly makes room for this specialist, the GNP. Increasingly she is becoming an integral part of the efforts toward quality care for America's elderly.

Who else cares for your parent?

3) The Administrator

Like the marker on a thermostat, it is the administrator who sets the warmth—or chill—the overall tone of a nursing home. Get to know him or her. Is he visible, respected, approachable? Or, isolated in his office, is he wedded to his calculator, typewriter, and telephone?

Mr. Voss is one administrator the residents admire. Entering into the lives of his "guests," as he calls them, he knows each one by name, keeps open the lines of communication among staff, residents, and community. He will dismiss any employee who fails to provide the kind of care that he would expect for his own parent.

In his nursing home, Mr. Voss is keen about "sensitivity training." Each new employee is required to assume the role of a patient for twenty-four hours before he or she is hired, a practice that gives valuable perspective on how it feels to be lifted out of bed, to remain for hours in a wheelchair, to be fed, to be ignored, to be the recipient of good care and much caring. Mr. Voss took this idea from a California community where legislators and commissioners tried it. Their reactions ran the gamut from amazement to sheer dismay as, for example, from their wheelchairs, they couldn't reach a water fountain or light switch or could not maneuver a trip to the restroom. Their experience resulted in many changed attitudes and in redesign of certain parts of the facility.

Mr. Voss knows that there is no such thing as a good nursing home that is not backed by the strong winds of community support. To strengthen the link between his home and the townspeople, he often speaks to civic, school, and church groups and releases periodic reports about the home to TV, radio, and the newspapers. He is in touch with the community college, to bring in life-long learning for his residents; in addition, he is in touch with the music school, and with the parks and recreation department, which is designing a special area for persons in wheelchairs to congregate for picnics. Mr. Voss has enlisted the help of an outside public-relations adviser to enhance strong contacts that contribute to the development of mutual understanding and good will between his nursing facility and the outlying area.

"A deadend home, a 'wayside station to the grave,' is not for us," says Mr. Voss. He hosts art shows in the lounge. Visitors are guided around the gallery of paintings by certain local residents. He encourages clients to hold bazaars for the community, to sell their own handmade products. His imagination soars as he turns his facility into a Center for Living. And I suspect that he approves of something novel that happens each summer at the Byron Health Care Center in Fort Wayne, Indiana. They rent a balloon. Eager residents (as many as will fit) are wheeled into the basket, to be lifted into the air for a view of the area. Talk about a center for living—summer hay-rides and beer parties, for example, are some of the invigorating surprises provided for by a caring administrator and his efficient staff. "As long as our clients have one more day to live," says Mr. Voss, "we'll see to it, wherever possible, that they live it to the fullest."

There came a day when another administrator, Mrs. Anderson, demonstrated her creativity. She learned that a local church group needed five hundred envelopes to be addressed and stuffed. "Why not enlist the aid of our residents?" she suggested. And so, amid sounds of delight, some of her residents gathered together, buckled down to work, and in four hours the job was done. Noting their renewed zest for life, Mrs. Anderson phoned a reporter. "Bring your camera," she requested. The next day, the scene made the local news. Excitedly pointing out their own faces, "There I am!" went the cry, or "There's Bessie—and there's Bob!" And the residents joked about having become famous.

This was not "busy-busy" work. This was the exhilaration of feeling needed—of swimming, once again as when they were younger—in the mainstream of society. The feeling is carried over again and again in this geriatric home, especially when residents create dolls and stuffed animals for hospitalized children and when they deliver these gifts personally, often handing them out from wheelchairs.

A wise administrator flings wide the gates, lets the public in. He believes in a strong volunteer corps for his facility, people to do things *with* not *for* others. He quotes Judge Brandeis: "What America needs is not to do things for people, but to *keep open the paths* which let them do things for themselves." More on this idea in chapter 10, "For Your Parent, Life More Abundant."

Thank you, Mr. Voss and Mrs. Anderson. You are right for your job. Thank you for making yourselves available to family members who need to talk to you about their special concerns. But alas! You have your counterpart. Introducing Mr. Briggs . . . .

Now here's one administrator who knows the name of at least one of his clients. He knows Jonathan. Why him in particular? Because Jonathan stamps out cigarette butts on the lounge carpet. On one occasion, Mr. Briggs was discovered communicating with a resident—this one—but hardly utilizing the gentle Voss approach.

A busy man, this Mr. Briggs. He owns four other nursing homes and two liquor stores. He commutes by Cadillac from his posh suburban estate. His nursing-home clients are poorly clothed, fed, housed. His facility is continuously being cited as substandard. This administrator sets his thermostat at "Chilly. Depressing."

In observing nursing facilities around the country, either as employee or researcher, I have encountered good administrators but also wild-and-woolly ones. How can one forget Mrs. Smyth, that law-and-order lady, who commanded one of those geriatric barracks? Her facility always passed inspections with flying colors. Immaculate. However, sorely afflicted with top-sergeant syndrome, Miss Efficiency cracked the hup-two-three-four whip, told you when to breathe in and when to breathe out. With clients, staff, and relatives, she was as popular as a boa constrictor.

In the nursing home where your parent lives, does the administrator receive credit for a job well done? Has he or she earned it? Here we must ask, "Why, over the years, has not a *qualified* administrator been required for *every* nursing home? Why, indeed, has such a person been as scarce as hen's teeth when it comes to awareness of the psychosocial needs of clients?" Can we pin this down?

Although the American College of Nursing Home Administrators displays the slogan "Ars, Virtus, Caritas," which captures the flavor of Academe, this organization is made up of only a small percentage of college graduates. In 1974, Samuel Levy, director of the Massachusetts state licensing program, found that only eighteen percent of that state's administrators had completed college, twenty-nine percent were high-school dropouts, and one percent had received no formal training at all. Since then, have these figures improved?

In June, 1977, I spotchecked that same state. Yes, things had improved. Twenty-seven percent of administrators had completed college, eleven and one-half percent had completed high school, and twelve percent were high-school dropouts. But this does not tell the whole tale. Fifty percent of the administrators who were questioned (in the same mail with license-renewal applications) ignored the questionnaire. Further, for many states, regulations provide only minimal requirements for the position. For example, as of this writing, the only requirements in one midwestern state are that (a) the applicant be over twenty-one; (b) the applicant be of "good character" (whatever that means); and (c) the applicant be a high-school graduate.

In the past, attempts to upgrade the position of nursing-home administrator through stiffer requirements have failed, due largely to roadblocks set up by certain nursing-home associations themselves. For example, a New York administrator was fired because he tried to push for tight peer-review controls. But the good news? Today, some states are moving toward at least two years, others toward four years, of college as a requisite for this key position.

Increasingly, the public hopes to see seminars for administrators which deal adequately not only with cost containment, budgets, and "optimum occupancy," but also with the psychosocial concerns of the elderly and with the broader arenas of gerontology. For example, let us consider the 1981 educational offerings for adminstrators by the American College of Nursing Home Administrators. Of the fifty seminars listed, only four deal directly with these important "human condition" aspects of the geriatric field. Lacking this foundation, how can a captain be expected to steer the ship on a straight course?

Today, we are beginning to see an increase in the attendance by administrators at regional and national gerontology conventions. These are the leaders who are beginning to set the thermostat ever higher—demanding quality care, hiring quality, competent personnel.

Who else cares for your parent?

4) The Social Worker

A pity! Here is a professional who frequently must prove his or her worth to the medical and nursing staffs. I recall one social worker, Mrs. Green, worth her weight in gold, who drove two hundred miles to address a physicians' breakfast seminar in Nebraska. Empty seats greeted her. Though disappointed, she told me, "This is not the first time. I will simply carry on with my job of improving morale among patients, staff, and families in the facility where I work. It is bringing about better cooperation among these groups." Then she added, "At first, doctors were skeptical of my usefulness, feeling that whatever I do, they do, and do it better. But soon they noted the changes a social worker can effect in a hospital or nursing facility. Today, in our medical care center, doctors put their arms around me and admit they cannot do without us!"

I asked Mrs. Green to explain her work. She told of a depressed woman who refused to join in activities, refused most of her food, spoke to no one. "I spent time with her," she said, "and learned that she was worried sick over a north window back home which she feared might not have been securely locked. I sent my son to check. He reported that all windows were locked tight. Given this information, the patient perked up, regained her appetite, began to socialize. It was as simple as that. But it took a social worker to spend time with her—time unavailable to the busy staff, to uncover the problem."

When we see how many caseloads social workers carry, we marvel at their achievements.

Competent social workers are indispensable members of any up-to-date rehabilitation team for the chronically ill, because *they give the entire health-care team a better understanding of the patient and his social and emotional environment.* Social workers help the patient and family accept illness and disability, help them with problems precipitated by this condition, encourage optimal utilization of medical care. What else does a social worker do? He or she helps the individual achieve his fullest capabilities, encourages development of new resources for unmet social service needs, encourages more effective use of hospital beds for the acutely ill through utilization of other community resources for the chronically ill when hospital care is no longer needed, and takes part in studies that will contribute to improved patient care and health programs in the community.

To sum up, the social worker helps the patient or nursing-home resident to find a satisfactory solution or adjustment to physical, emotional, and economic problems by exploring those areas, both present and past, that affect the patient's total health condition and by offering support to both patient and family.

Sometimes, the social worker is the only link an institutionalized person has with the outside world—especially when relatives live far away or are unable to visit often. Get to know the social worker. This person is your liaison—among you, your parent, and the nursing home—ready and competent to assist you professionally in many ways.

We have talked about some of the nursing-home staff. Others on the staff, vital to the effort, will be honored as you read further in this book. At this point, however, we must discuss briefly a serious aspect of care which involves all staff members. *Be aware of your parent's need for privacy.* As an old German proverb reminds us, "A hedge between keeps friendships green." How does the staff uphold this need?

The Gift of Privacy*

Privacy? A must for your mother.

Look into Mrs. Jones's room. Whew! A ceaseless frenzy of activity! From morning till night her room is invaded by aides making beds or bedpanning her roommate. The lab man wants a "sample." The housekeeper shines the furniture. Windows are washed. The janitor has a job to do. The nurse passes meds. Noisy visitors of Mrs. Jones's roommate compete with sounds from the hall—call bells, telephones. And how about that mumbling woman dropping in, mistaking this room for her own? Just as things start to quiet down, the student-nurse

---
*Article by Nancy Fox, originally published in *Geriatric Care*, April, 1981. Eyeman Publications, Inc., Box 3577, Reno, NV 89505.

group enters, ready to "guinea-pig" her. Is there no rest for the weary? Oh, oh, now it's that roommate again. This time, after concluding her coughing spell, she dials the radio—and what does our Mrs. Jones get? Garish commercials. (Does Mrs. Jones need new spark-plugs, a diamond that is forever, a Hart Schaffner Marx suit?) Now it's that roaring evangelist. "*Must* I put up with *him?*" moans Mrs. Jones. "I'm going crazy. No privacy."

Privacy is that oft-neglected patients' right and an essential ingredient for mental health. At times we must be alone to find order, to make sense out of our existence, to maintain a sense of self. "For it is in solitude," said Robert Lintner, "that the works of hand, heart, and mind are always conceived, and in solitude that individuality must be affirmed."

When privacy is constantly invaded, one tends to withdraw communication—as a turtle draws into its shell. Does this explain in part why some residents refuse to join in activities? Much privacy is lost in the routine of congregate living. Staff and residents must try to provide as much privacy for a patient as is humanly possible.

Is the nursing-home staff aware of this need for your mother? Do they knock before entering her room? Do they respect her diaries, albums, personal letters? Do they allow her, if she is able, to open her own mail? Do they respect the modesty of an older person, keeping her covered until the moment she steps into her bath? Of course, you will see those privacy-curtains—intended to seclude her bed area when attendants or doctors give treatments. But the question is: Are these curtains actually drawn when needed?

Ninety-five year old Mrs. Warner's privacy and modesty needs were not being met. Therein lay the cause of an eruption, an inevitable clash of personalities. Unless staff understands the background of each client, it cannot give quality care. This particular staff knew nothing about Mrs. Warner, although there it was, documented in the social history section of her chart.

Mrs. Warner was born into a sedate minister's family. Reared in the Victorian era—that "never-without-a hat," that white gloves and parasol era—she was known for her perfect manners, gentleness of speech, and correct attire. She was and is "every inch a lady." Staff, however, showed no interest in learning about her, as a person. Aides were not briefed on her strict background. And so, they could not, would not grant her one simple request.

On the surface, the problem seemed small. All Mrs. Warner wanted was to be "correctly attired," both inside and out. She was appalled when, each morning, aides refused to help her don her panties. "A lady simply does not go without them," she haughtily informed her caretakers. But they insisted: "It's easier to take you to the bathroom without them. Who cares anyway, who's to know?"

Helpless, Mrs. Warner feels that her dignity has been undermined, that her decision-making days are over, her privacy violated. Further, while she is in the bathroom, must they always leave the door open? Staff scolds her for her "silly" demands. And this person, throughout her lifetime known as a dignified, soft-spoken aristocrat, is viewed in the nursing home as a crotchety, demanding, "impossible" crank.

Other geriatric homes, however, are sensitive to the importance of privacy for any human being. Quiet places are accessible for residents—garden pathways; retreats; a library where silence is maintained; the chapel; little soundproof cubicles for reading, writing, meditation, or a confidential rendezvous.

"The human animal needs freedom from intrusion," says Phyllis McGinley. "He needs a little privacy, quite as much as he needs understanding or vitamins or exercise or praise." May your mother find peace of mind through needed privacy—that gift all the more treasured if ever it has been withheld.

And now, family, how do you size up the staff? Do you note friendly rapport between staff and patients? Staff and relatives? Staff and staff?

You have met this team, those who are there to draw a circle of love around your parent. Remember, there are still others — the faithful "invisibles," who oil the wheels of the institution — those from the laundry, dietary, housekeeping, clerical, and maintenance departments. All must pull together. To provide quality care, it takes a full team.

Quality care? Not just a flowery term, but the specific goal of a good home, attainable through competence and positive expectations of the entire staff — expectations not only for themselves as health-care providers, but for the rehabilitation potential of each resident. Quality care is only an empty boast on a public-relations brochure unless it is reflected in the care your mother receives. Quality care eases loneliness, provides social and therapeutic involvement, and offers incentive to live. Should you settle for less?

Who cares for your mother? Not the fly-by-night in need of a temporary job. Let it be those who bring alive the words of the Prophet: "All work is empty, save where there is love."

Nothing is harder than the softness of indifference.
Montoya

6
Is This Senility Necessary?*

Although only a small percentage (some experts put the figure at 5 percent) of America's sixty-and-over population suffers chronic, irreversible, incurable organic brain syndromes, now known as Alzheimer's Disease,** countless others in nursing homes may be victims of what I have called "man-made senility." Torsos tilting sideways, eyes glassy, mouths drooling—do you think that in old age this is inevitable?

You have heard of man-made limbs, man-made other body

---

*Parts of this chapter were published originally in "Northwest Magazine," the Sunday supplement of the newspaper *The Oregonian*, 20 January 1980. Used by permission.

**The Johns Hopkins Department of Psychiatry has established a psycho-geriatric health team of psychiatrists, psychiatric nurses, psychologists, social workers, and other geriatric specialists who are involved in Alzheimer's Disease education, research, and patient care, as well as in developing family-support systems. Increasingly, around the United States and Canada, this kind of research is being conducted, for, as yet, the cause or causes of this disease are unknown.

parts, but this idea of man-made senility, I suspect, is new to you. In this chapter we will look at this creeping symptom which can subdue any nursing-home client unless staff uses extreme caution.

Need you stand by helplessly? Not if you watch for the three warning flags: Infantizing, Over-rest, and Oversedation.

Infantizing

"Are we ready for our little pill, Ducky?"
"How do we feel this morning?"
"Here, let's put on our bib, shall we?"

These are samples of infantizing, that is, the pressuring of an adult into a state of infancy. The use of "we" rather than "you" robs a person of his or her identity. Talking down to clients contributes to their low self-esteem. A federal study on long-term care facilities reports, "Surveyors noted that in a large number of facilities, patients' dependency attitudes were reinforced continuously by the manner in which staff addressed them—often as though speaking to a child."

Reader, so that you may recognize this practice and prevent it from affecting your mother, note some further examples:

Mrs. Park, a retired teacher, can tell you about infantizing. Without her consent, the staff calls her "Amy." A dress protector is tied around her neck, but they call it a "bib." A box of Pampers sits in plain view on her dresser. As though Mrs. Park cannot understand English, employees refer to her in her presence as "a difficult case." Her body lies exposed while staff changes her linens. And when Mrs. Park sometimes puts up mild resistance, aides shake their heads, wondering "why Amy acts so childish."

Diapers, bibs, baby-talk—the only thing missing, sighs Mrs. Park, is a rattle. Because of poor health and diminished sight and hearing, she has gradually been reduced to the status

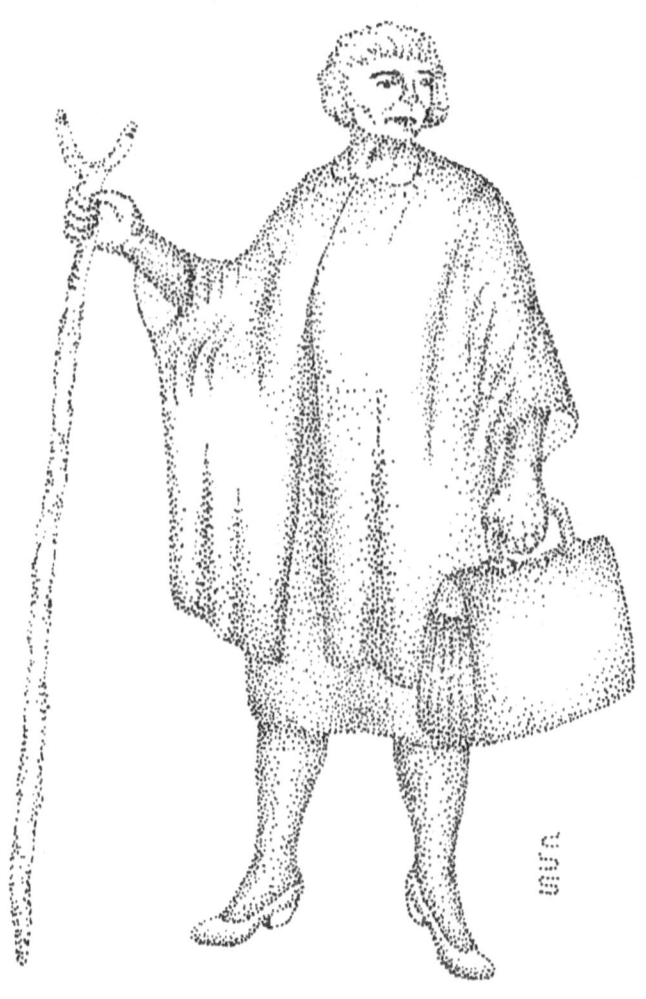

Margaret Meade, believing in her own late-life potential, kept teaching and working till the end of her days. She walked with a tall walking stick, which was given her by a tribe among whom she lived in New Guinea.

of an infant. For the sake of institutional efficiency, she has been molded into a caricature of a human being.

"Treat me like a child," exclaims her roommate, "and I will stamp my feet to demand attention and throw my food on the floor! But then, of course, society will label me 'senile.'"

Across the hall, Mr. Purdy tosses in the night. He longs for a glass of warm milk, but refuses to ring his call bell. He already knows what the response will be: "If we'd eaten all our din-din last night, we wouldn't be hungry at this ungodly hour, would we?"

In another facility, Mr. McGuire tackles the "opposition" head on. Into his room trips the well-meaning young nursing aide. "Are we ready for our bath?" she squeals.

"Yes!" bellows the disgusted old gentleman. "We are ready. Let's jump in!"

The staff member who infantizes older persons may be unaware that this practice can be humiliating to the long-lived person. As a relative, you can gently remind the well-meaning staff that "Mother prefers adult-to-adult communication."

Another contributor to man-made senility is called, quite simply, "rest." That is, over-rest.

Over-rest

"Rest!" you exclaim. "Come now, what's wrong with rest? We all need it. My parent, especially."

Would you believe that rest, this seemingly harmless pastime, can demoralize a person if taken in endless doses? The problem is that you-need-your-rest syndrome is sanctioned by too many "rest" homes. *Too much* rest. No end of rest. As a relative, you may need to monitor the amount of rest your parent receives. Why? Because gerontologists tell us today that one of the most dangerous treatments for the aged is enforced inactivity. Passivity and immobility can and often do lead to a rapid decline in health—even to a total disability. "Nonsense," you protest. "Nobody ever died of rest!" Oh, no? If he could, the late Mr. Carr would disagree. What happened to him happens to too many nursing-home clients.

Arriving at the facility, Mr. Carr is introduced to his roommate and to the staff. After that there is not much communication, for repeatedly he is told: "Time to rest. Doctor's orders." And so he gets it—plenty of rest. Mornings he lolls on his bed. Afternoons he dozes in his chair. Lights out at 7:00 p.m. After only one week, he sees a bleak future for himself.

Months pass. Lack of physical and mental stimulation take their toll. With his interest in life drained, Mr. Carr now qualifies for membership in the "Seniles Club." Due to lack of sensory stimulation, he forgets easily, mutters to himself. Due to poor muscle tóne, his bladder control is gone; he soils himself and gets frequently scolded. Time now for Mr. Carr to join that catheterized, bed-ridden, faceless throng—victims of the plenty-of-rest school of thought. Soon he develops bladder infection, perhaps bedsores. Finally, he is hospitalized for pneumonia, treated, and released. His latest medical orders . . . You guessed it . . . "Plenty of rest." "Yes," agrees the staff, "he needs his rest."

Three days later he gets the best rest there is, the most perfect rest known to man. He's resting in peace. A sheet is pulled over his head.

Positive that they have provided tender loving care—in fact, unaware of mismanagement—the medical and nursing teams make the comment, "Oh, well, Harry's better off now. There was nothing to live for."

Although you as a lay person have an inkling about what happens to minds and bodies when all this resting goes on, health professionals can sometimes forget that this may result in dulling of the intellect, increased dependency, metabolic imbalances, circulatory deterioration, mental confusion, loss of muscular strength and endurance, deterioration of the cerebrovascular system and, finally, loss of self-esteem. The list can go on and on.

Although today some doctors and nurses are shortening

those interminable rest periods in nursing homes (they've been cutting down on *hospital* bedrest for years), there is still resistance. "Why change the routine?" the long-term care staff complains. "Old people have worked hard all their lives; they need their rest."

Another contributor to man-made senility is the medically prescribed tranquilizer.

Oversedation

Extend your antennae. With eyes, ears, and nostrils, tune in—not just to observe, but to scrutinize the facility. Peek into remote corners. Take the elevator to the uppermost floors, if it is a large building, to see if certain "hopeless" clients may be stashed away, out of sight, out of the public mind. In some homes, particularly in large cities, what might you find? Patients not recognizing their families. Heads flopping into supper trays. Bodies tied to chairs. Voices mumbling, wailing, cackling, screaming.

Ravaging disease, of course, can cause some of these conditions. Our immediate concern, however, is: how many of these unfortunates are paying the penalty of months—indeed, of years—of mismanagement? How many were infantized, over-rested, oversedated? Ask yourself the burning question: "Is this senility necessary?" How many of these patients, with proper therapeutic intervention, might have been spared such an existence?

Each year in American nursing homes, millions of tranquilizers are used. "An effective way," said one senator, "to put people in a position where they will not complain or demand services." An effective way, we may add, to hasten brain sluggishness—or man-made senility.

Mrs. Korman has just been added to the list of those who are chemically restrained. Why? Because she loved to dance. She was full of vitality, walked all over the home. Staff was never quite sure where she was or what she was doing. Consequently, they informed the doctor that they couldn't stand it any longer and asked whether he might not "prescribe a tranquilizer." And so he did. A pity the nursing staff itself, in this case, lacked the imagination to come up with an alternative plan to make Mrs. Korman's life meaningful.

Auschwitz was perhaps the most cruel of the Hitler prison camps. Many of our elderly, living in an Auschwitz of their own, are prisoners of altered states of consciousness. Says Dr. Alexander Simon, medical director of the Langley-Porter Neuro-Psychiatric Institute in San Francisco, "*Once you start* giving any kind of sedative that has an effect on the metabolism of the brain, you may precipitate an acute confusional state, especially likely in aged patients. *This can easily be mistaken for senility.*"

"Once you start"—this is your cue, relative of a patient. Obtain complete information as to what medications your parent is receiving, as discussed in chapter 3, "A Mighty Fortress, the Family." It is well known that for every drug consumed, including aspirin, there are side-effects. Each new drug added to a patient's medications increases the potential for reaction. And so, what about such reactions?

Now you and I are not doctors or pharmacologists, but neither are we dummies. Sometimes even the patient is aware of the lunacy of this sort of thing and spits the stuff out.

This is not to deny that for your parent there may be the possible need and value of certain drugs in certain amounts. Says pharmacologist Edward Brady, M.S., associate dean of the School of Pharmacy at the University of Southern California, "The concern is that drugs can stupify, injure, cause waste and harmful problems that are preventable. Nursing-home residents on tranquilizers often suffer reactions that require hospitalization. As if that were not anguish enough, thousands experience drug reaction while in the hospital, thus doubling their length of stay."

And here, our concern extends beyond the nursing home. What about the powerful drug corporations who spend billions of dollars annually to advertise their products? Clever ads blur the judgment of many a doctor, appealing to "ease of management" or "social control," rather than to the therapeutic needs of the patient. One ad, for a long time found in professional journals, dramatized in bold red letters the "tantrums" of "senile psychosis"—finally consumer advocate groups protested. In that same ad one notes eighty-three lines of fine print, mentioning, as required by law, the possible adverse effects of the drug—everything from jaw twitchings to disturbance of cardiac rhythm to sudden death. "Give Brand 'X'," said one ad, "to benefit all concerned—staff, family, and patient." And there in the ad one saw the accompanying picture of a winsome, brightly attired great-grandmother, oh, so joyously drugged and relaxed!

Some nurses, however, find it difficult to remain joyous and relaxed, knowing that, for their patients, indiscriminate doses are being prescribed. Increasingly they are speaking out, assuming active responsibility in discussing this with their doctors and Geriatric Nurse Practitioners. If you suspect overdrugging in your parent, speak to the head nurse, who, well aware that today we live in an era of wholesale "brain-blowing," may be working to counter the trend.

Because of physiological changes, the elderly cannot absorb drugs as rapidly as younger people. Dr. Eric Pfeiffer, of Duke University Medical Center, notes, "We must be extraordinarily cautious in the use of drugs in the elderly, who have delicately balanced systems which can easily be derailed by a number of drugs which have proved beneficial in younger patients."

Another question: What about the legality of overdrugging? Recently a district judge ruled that excessive use of tranquilizers may infringe on patients' rights.

These, then, are some of the contributors to man-made senility which, in the well-run, well-staffed nursing home, you will not have to contend with. Over-rest, oversedation. Bodies drooping, eyes glassy, mouth gaping—no! These sights are *not* inevitable with old age. If you suspect that your parent may be subjected to one or all of these avoidable conditions, investigate. This is your legal right. It is not always patients' behaviors which need adjusting; sometimes it is the philosophy and behavior of the staff which must be changed.

Friends and relatives of the institutionalized, you have a job to do. Help stamp out man-made senility. Keep a watchful eye, so that your parent is not exposed to approaches that guarantee mental deterioration. Be on guard. Speak out where you find abuses, or where you note that, as Nurse Frances Storlie observed: "Cruelty can be so subtle that even the cruel don't recognize it."

You have been alerted to three contributors to senility. There are others, beyond the scope of this book, which should at least be mentioned. We refer to the physiological aspects of confusion, as pointed out by Dr. Mary Wolanin, professor emeritus of the University of Arizona. Among others, she mentions iron and calcium deficiency, hypo- and hyperthermia, and impaction—all of which are preventable and curable. In particular, let us dwell for a moment on hypothermia.

Does your mother complain of cold hands and feet? Does she feel cold to the touch, although not shivering? There are other symptoms as well. Accidental hypothermia (the dipping of body temperature below normal and on down to 94 degrees or lower) can be dangerous. Victims are often those with chronic illness, especially diseases of the veins and arteries, and those taking certain drugs for anxiety, nausea, and agitation. In Britain, it is estimated that up to ten thousand elderly people die each year of hypothermia.

Be alert, then, to the room temperatures of the home, and see that Mother has plenty of blankets to keep her warm. Perhaps an aging person is labeled a "chronic complainer" when actually he or she *is* cold.

You and your parent are fortunate, indeed, if you are satisfied with the care provided—if you find no reason to confront the home authorities with the question: "Is this senility necessary?"

There is no such thing as a good nursing home unless, through rehabilitation and social involvement, it eases loneliness and offers incentive to live.

7
Think Therapy

Is your mother receiving therapy? One or more kinds, on a daily basis? This can make the difference between progress and backsliding. Therapy often results in dramatic improvement of mental and physical functions. For the sake of your mother's well-being, this subject requires scrutiny.

Nursing facilities must depend upon and cooperate with the therapist, for what that person does lays the foundation for what the rest of the staff can do. When a therapist offers your parent hope and renewed mobility of mind, body, and spirit, the staff can proceed to build upon her individual care plan, pursuing newer, ever-bolder activities and objectives. In time, the enrichment of her life is the inevitable result. We bless the therapy team, not only for the way it changes attitudes toward illness, but for the gentle ways it brings new meaning to many lives.

The nursing home that does not emphasize therapy is a ship without a rudder; its passengers flounder aimlessly, their destinations obscure. We use the word *emphasize* because *every* nursing home is legally required to offer physical- and occupational-therapy services. But does this mean that every resident automatically receives these services? Is your mother benefiting from any kind of therapy?

Remember that when you were shopping for a nursing home the administrator proudly pointed out the fancy therapy rooms and equipment? And that at the time, you assumed that all of these benefits would naturally befall your own loved one? Has this materialized for her on a daily basis? What about weekends, as well, when a part-time therapist should be taking over the job? Or, still chanting that old "short-of-help" tune, is the staff of the home becalmed for forty-eight hours, imposing a dead halt on these essential services?

According to a 1975 report from the Department of Health, Education and Welfare (now known as the Department of Health and Human Services), we learned that in U.S. nursing homes:

> 70 percent need, *but are not getting*, physical therapy
> 89 percent need, *but are not getting*, occupational therapy
> 90 percent need, *but are not getting*, speech therapy

These figures could well apply to the 1980s, in many geriatric facilities, whose activity rooms are not fully utilized. The competent activities director plans a program, ideally designed to enhance quality of life—a broad scope of activities which have meaning for the individual.

In the past, the responsibility has fallen on the director, but today, we know that he or she cannot do it all. Staff must help to motivate residents to participate. It takes the team which employs loving approaches, consistent invitations, and gentle persuasion to bring residents out of their cubicles into the activity rooms—out of isolation and back into a life of greater creativity. And staff must respect the wishes of those who may never wish to participate, but prefer to work alone, to meditate, to compose a poem, a song, or something which he or she does better when alone. As one resident put it, "Potholders are not for everyone!" You, the relative, can be supportive of your parent, as far as activities go; and you can help the activities director to understand better the wishes, preferences, and background of your mother. In time, she may join a group and continue doing those things which used to bring her pleasure, pride, and personal satisfaction.

If your parent is not included in the therapy or rehabilitation programs, question the head nurse. If you are told that the doctor did not order it, make an appointment to see him or her. Remind him of Title One, Section Four, of the Older Americans' Act, which calls for "full, restorative services for those who require institutionalization."

Why, if such services are not needed, was she admitted to this costly facility? This is a nursing home, a "convalescent center," isn't it? Again, remind yourself, *it is not a hotel!* Therefore, with no extra billing to the client, therapy and rehabilitation should be included in each one's daily schedule as automatically as she gets bed and board. It is ironic, isn't it, that a nursing home ad will often boast, "Therapy available"? Of course! Why shouldn't it be? That statement is comparable to that of a restaurant that advertises: "Food available."

And family, while you are on this path, you might remind the doctor, also, to read the preamble to Title One of the Older Americans' Act:

> The Congress of the United States hereby finds . . . that, in keeping with the traditional concept of the inherent dignity of the individual in our democratic society, the older people of our nation are entitled to, . . . and [it] is the joint . . . duty and responsibility of the States to assist older people to secure, equal opportunity to the full and free enjoyment of the following objectives . . .

And it goes on to mention, among other objectives, those "full, restorative services."

Therapy, restorative services—these are the right of all institutionalized persons. For your parent, this need must not be ignored.

Why is therapy important? What does it accomplish?

Therapy builds upon a person's strengths of mind, body, and spirit. It enhances dignity, self-esteem. Mother comes to feel that someone cares enough to make these efforts on her behalf. "I'm worth it!" she says. "There is potential for me to function on a higher plane. The therapist believes in me, and so I believe in myself, and I will cooperate."

If Mother is receiving therapy, fine. She is in the hands of highly skilled professionals who reach into the heart, draw out the goodness, the life-spark that may be lying dormant. Salvaging a sense of worth, **conveying a message of caring**, the therapist works to restore your mother to her highest potential and capabilities.

Besides physical, occupational, and recreational therapy, or included in these categories, are many other kinds of therapies. In the long-term home, there should be evidence of these other therapies such as family therapy, music therapy,* dance, poetry, wine therapy (if your parent approves), puppet therapy, and horticultural therapy—as well as many other kinds designed to help reverse various medical or psychological impairments. To describe a few:

Milieu Therapy: This transforms a client's environment into a therapeutic community, that is, he participates in his own care and treatment, takes responsibility for himself and often for others. For example, tying this in with the poetry class, he regains or maintains his ability to select and read a poem to others, may even help to conduct the class. He may also be able to wheel a less independent patient outdoors for some sunshine.

Resocialization Therapy: This is designed to improve mental attitudes and socialization. A group gathers, and reminiscing is encouraged. For many clients, this is valuable.

---

*Recommended: *Music in Geriatric Care* (New York: St. Martin's Press) by Ruth Bright, music therapist, New South Wales Health Department, Australia.

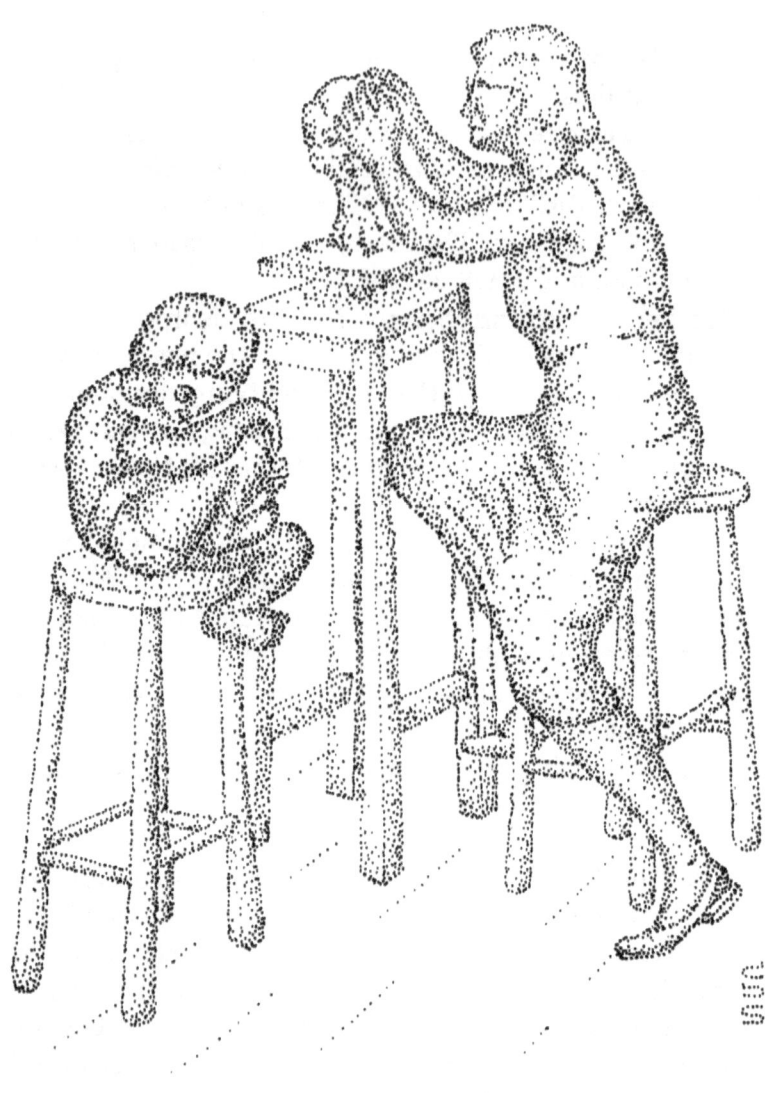

"I always wanted to try my hand at something creative so I joined a clay sculpture class at the home. Now my grandson poses for me once a week. It's not just mindless busy work. It's a challenge and I'm learning. I've awakened dormant abilities when I have the time to use them and I feel better."

They are reminded of the old days "when I was someone important," or "when I was needed by my family and community." Recently, a hard-of-hearing resident told how he was elected a county official. Bursting his buttons with pride, he passed around a snapshot of his handsome young self, standing alongside his red Buick. Atop the vehicle were blazoned the words: "Bill Devon, County Commissioner."

Reality Orientation Therapy: This brings to the confused client a better awareness of day-to-day facts and an increased awareness of wanting to do things for one's self. He is asked—or is told—the time of day, the date, the month, where he used to live, the names of his children, and so on. Signs are posted in large letters to remind him of the day's activities. For such a resident, it is important that the entire staff participate in his reality orientation, which can be practiced during tubbings, manicures, meals—indeed, during any time of contact with him. Without this kind of therapy, the resident may slip further into isolation, into a fanciful world of his own. Ask the therapist about Validation/Fantasy Therapy (see Appendix, page 168).

Prayer Therapy: Was your parent once active in church or synagogue? Does she miss the involvement, the frequent services and sacrifices to the glory of her God? Even if the priest, rabbi, or minister occasionally drops in to visit the flock, is this sufficient spiritual support? Prayer therapy may be a comforting intervention. Regardless of the religious or nonreligious beliefs of the staff, here they focus solely on the religious needs of the resident—interceding when your parent sends forth a spiritual SOS or, better, *before* a crisis arises. To alleviate her anguish, a staff member holds her hand, prays with her, affirms her spiritual need, puts on her chart: "Pray with her PRN (when needed)." For when a religiously-oriented client, perhaps your own mother, feels heavy-laden, is there any medication or any therapy more powerful than prayer?

Ask the head nurse if, in this home, the in-service training includes how to recognize and help fulfill the spiritual needs of residents. For, as Mrs. Dorothy McCool, an Oregon head nurse told me, "If the goal is truly *total* care—the integration of body, mind, and spirit therapies—of the three, *spiritual* care for many may well be the most valuable therapy of all."

Pet Therapy: For residents who are depressed and feel useless, this kind of therapy has worked wonders to raise morale. One humane society in Colorado takes its "Pet-Mobile" twice a month to visit at four nursing homes, and the response is a joy to behold! One nursing-home administrator allows the pets in the home, others prefer to have them visit with residents on the grounds surrounding the home. In any case, the therapeutic benefits for those who love animals, and are, in return, loved by the pets, is of inestimable value.*

Remotivation Therapy: This stimulates the unmotivated and encourages social participation in arts, crafts, movies, singing—whatever offers human contact. As Dr. Robert Butler explains it, the technique consists of the following five steps, used with groups of from five to fifteen residents:

1) The climate of acceptance—establishing a warm, friendly relationship within the group.
2) A bridge to reality—reading of objective poetry, current events, and other similar materials.
3) Sharing the world—development of this topic through planned, objective questions, the use of props, and so on.
4) An appreciation of the work of the world—designed to stimulate the residents' thinking about the work of the world in relation to themselves.
5) The climate of appreciation—expression of enjoyment at getting together, and so on.

Within the above framework, this kind of therapy tries to

---

*Some non-paying guests of the Lewiston Health Care Center in Idaho include a cat, a dog, and a parakeet. This makes for a homelike atmosphere.

discover what activities a resident enjoyed earlier in life and then encourages him toward those same goals, as much as possible, within the nursing-home setting.

Psychotherapy: This is the least available kind of therapy to older people, whether confined or residing in the community, but one which should be part of any therapeutic relationship. Says Dr. Robert Butler, head of the National Institute on Aging, "Psychotherapy deals with losses, grief, bodily dysfunction, and so forth. The older person needs a secure confidant." Dr. Butler believes that older people deserve it and are as good candidates for successful psychotherapy as are those of any other age group.

We now draw special attention to an essential form of therapy—**speech therapy**. And we ask: Why is it that so many administrators fail to employ speech therapists?

According to Alice Swallum, a South Dakota speech therapist, many therapists in the United States remain unemployed. We believe that (because the College of Nursing-Home Administrators stresses fiscal management in their workshops) this need has gone unrecognized or at least its importance has been minimized. A full-time speech therapist in every nursing home? Costly? Yes. But if the client comes first, could there not be rethinking of priorities?

What devastating frustration is felt by a patient, perhaps after a stroke, when he cannot express himself? (A glass of orange juice was thrown in my face by such a patient, frantic because she could not make herself understood.) Physicians might consider the compelling case for speech therapy which can do wonders for many to alleviate this feeling of helplessness. Professionals know that when early treatment is initiated, partial or total rehabilitation can be possible. The hiring of one or more speech therapists could make the difference in many a long-term care home between joy and despair, and yes, even the will to live.

Your parent pays good money to live here. Unquestionably,

services such as speech therapy should be included for those who need it, particularly in the light of a statement made by a Wichita psychologist, John Valusek: "It is immoral to interfere with the potential of others."

What about the therapy which comes through the efforts of the **activities director?** The goal here is not just busy-busy pastimes but, insofar as possible, to turn dependence and apathy into self-determination and activism. If we are talking about continuation of growth, the program should be responsive to the holistic or whole needs of each participant—providing a satisfactory emotional response, together with physical and mental stimulation.

In some geriatric homes, I have noted excellent results, even personality changes, brought about by competent activities directors. The programs offered today, in certain homes, are a far cry, and a joyous one, from programs offered ten years ago. They take into consideration that it is not the *time* spent on activities that matters so much as the *meaning* that these tasks have for the resident and the extent of his or her wholehearted involvement.

Beauty Therapy: Beauty therapy? What's that? To demonstrate the value of this offering, let me paint for you a familiar picture. You women readers have probably experienced this yourselves in your home life.

The doorbell rings. The knocker pounds. What a shock! Here it is, early morning, and I'm looking like something the cat dragged in. Hair flying. Face puffy. Teeth as yet unbrushed. Mouth feels like cobwebs. Shabby slippers. Junky bathrobe, which, I swear, I was planning any day now to scrap!

But that knock? I flee to the kitchen. Yet the urgent sound forces me to return and open the door. (And all he wants—I could wring his neck—is for me to take his child to school!)

Hours later, convalescing from this ordeal, I begin to think about it—serious thoughts about that wheelchair patient I had recently visited. Mrs. Tallman had been stuffed into any old outfit and wore no makeup. Her hair was unbrushed. Hating herself, she apologized for her appearance. And I heard an aide remark: "We'll skip the tooth-brushing today, Dearie, I'm in a rush." (Meaning: "You're not worth it. I'm eager for my coffee-break.")

Does it matter how the institutionalized person looks, and what that person wears? For her morale, it matters intensely what Mother wears, how she looks. Clothing and appearance have a strong effect on how people feel about themselves. Confidence in personal appearance is essential to a sense of dignity and worth.*

Today's modern nursing facility provides a beauty parlor. But does every resident get to use it? Regularly? What about your parent, if she is bedbound, unable to be wheeled "down there"? Perhaps her need is all the greater for beauty therapy.

Today I thanked a young volunteer, Connie, who goes to a convalescent home to give facials. I had steered her to a patient who had recently fallen and who, when I last saw her, was depressed. *Of course* she was! Hair knotty. No makeup. Same old story. Connie makes these people feel like a million dollars. "Nancy," she says, "if you think facials bring joy to residents, imagine how their joy uplifts *me*!"

Do you remember the song, "I Feel Pretty"? Would a woman sing that song dressed as I—"Mrs. Dracula"—was on that dreadful morning? I think she'd have changed her tune to ask for, "Just One More Chance."

If beauty is in the eyes of the beholder, perhaps your mother needs to feel as "beholdable" as possible as long as she lives in a nursing home.

Mealtime: What could be more therapeutic than a sociable, nicely served, delicious dinner? In the home, how do you rate

---

*Recognizing this, the Sister Kenny Institute (Chicago Avenue at 27th, Minneapolis, MN 55407) has put out booklet #737, giving ideas for smart clothing for the handicapped, how to adapt clothing or revise patterns. Also it suggests clever use of scarves and other simple accessories to accentuate the positive.

this daily event in the eyes of your parent?

"Dinner is served!" The dining-room door swings open to a cluster of residents who have waited outside it for heaven-knows-how-long. They breathe a sigh of relief. "At last," murmurs one woman, "now we get to dine—highlight of my day!"

Family, you came here today to check out the meals in this home, to analyze staff attitudes, to observe in detail how this daily ritual is carried out. You join a foursome at one of the tables prettily set with fresh flowers.

In any good home, the goal of the nutrition program goes beyond merely balancing the nutrients. Meals are meant for taste, nostril, and eye appeal and especially for the benefits of relaxed sociability. (You trust that very few residents eat alone in their rooms, but you will check that out later.) This place, so far, seems all right, you think, as your mind wanders back to that other home you visited where meals were a disaster. Where nobody spoke a word. Where a sticky-sweet, garishly-colored jelly-like substance passed for salad, and where, noisily and hurriedly, plates of brown "slop" were plunked down before the residents. And that awful dessert—small slices of dehydrated white cake! And diluted, cool coffee. So now, what about *this* home?

Already you note the difference. By the manner in which the meal is served, your hopes rise. Pleasant, crispy-clean nurse-aides, interacting with residents and trained to serve graciously, seem to be enjoying their task. (It used to be that at Antoine's Restaurant in New Orleans, a busboy received seven years of training in the art of serving a meal before he was considered for the job of waiter.) In this home, there has surely been some careful training along these lines, for at once you get the message. Dinner is being served with care and pride.

Enter now Mrs. Walters, the registered dietitian, who is checking to make sure each resident is doing O.K., determined to make each one feel he or she is someone special. In command of the situation she asks, "Mr. Knobel, would you like rye bread or wheat?" or "Would you take your juice now or later, dear Mrs. Sills?"

Mrs. Walters allows for decision-making. It is her conviction that when individuality gives way to mass treatment, dignity is sacrificed. Here, no such sacrifice is imminent, it appears, as long as Mrs. Walters reigns "Queen of the Cuisine." Her meals carry the message: "We care about you—about your tastes, your feelings, about you, as a person." And here, the attitudes, even if the food were unpalatable, symbolize the quality of care to which this home is dedicated. Every dish, with its variety, texture, and color, is a work of art. And you notice that the portions are small—a subtle way of saying, "Have some more!"

Every dish a work of art? Look at that attractive appetizer, the half-grapefruit scalloped around the rim, with a maraschino cherry in the center. Or that sprig of fresh parsley decorating the ground sirloin patty. And those hot bran rolls served from a pretty basket. Not to mention those pink and green after-dinner mints—little creative touches requiring only moments of preparation, plus love and imagination, to enhance the experience of institutional dining.

Royal treatment, too, is accorded those residents on special diets. At their tables you notice sugarless cookies, salt-free relishes—appropriate yet tempting goodies. "Well, Mrs. Chalmers, are you enjoying your dinner?" asks Mrs. Gregory, the administrator, who has slipped in to show her interest. Like a mother hen, she hovers over a resident. (She knows each one by name—loves them all.)

Bare tables? Here at the Park Hill Home, perish the thought. Colorful clean cloths, although necessarily of plastic, look like real linen. And during dinner, you are dimly aware of the soft background music that eases tension and relaxes tired bodies. Nobody hurries. The staff glides about quietly and never will you hear what Mrs. Walters considers to be the cardinal culinary crime: the clattering of chinaware from the kitchen area.

Yes, dinner at this home means good food, good conversation, and leisurely enjoyment. And if, because of Mrs. Walters' workload and that of the dietary staff, the meals cannot quite be classified as "gourmet," even more important, they are served with love, each meal a special event. "Gracious dining" you could call it—something you hardly expected to find in an institution. Your preconceptions fly out the window. And you cannot help but smile—no, marvel—as you see the shine in those eyes at the approach of mealtime. No wonder the residents here perk up at the sound of those magic words, "Dinner is served!"

Let's now tour the kitchen. This one looks clean, well organized. It would have to be to provide such a meal as you have just enjoyed. Again, compare. What a contrast to the one in another home where you visited an elderly aunt. There, the patient was low man on the totem pole. That place was eventually closed down and no wonder. You remember the dented, damaged food cans, the unmopped kitchen floor, the meats that remained for hours on the counter (to the everlasting delight of the fly population). At that facility, turnover of cooks and kitchen helpers was appalling. You recall the evening when supper didn't appear. The evening wore on. Your aunt was "starving." The cook had quit. Dirty dishes were strewn all over. Discovering only unappetizing leftovers in the messy refrigerator, an aide rose to the occasion. And residents had quite a supper! She gave them all graham crackers and milk.

What, then, does it take, besides the dedication and imagination of a dietary staff, to maintain a good cuisine? As you tour that area, look for telltale signs. Do you note an abundance of fresh fruits and vegetables—including leafy green and yellow ones? Plenty of fresh milk, whole grain breads and cereals, brown rice, bran and other unrefined foods? Surely you will find no trace of that ghastly, artificial liquid that passes for orange juice and no processed or "convenience" foods—full of additives, preservatives. At the English Hills Home in Grand Rapids, Michigan, I experienced something unusual. In the interest of better nutrition, and with the hearty approval of residents, only decaffeinated coffee is served.

As you toured the kitchen area, you may have marveled at the planning it takes, not just for regular diets, but for the special ones—diets for the diabetic person, for those with dental or gastrointestinal ailments, or for those with allergies or certain dislikes or preferences. And you have asked what would be a good diet for your parent. It would depend upon both her health status and her own habits, making it an individual matter between her and her physician. (Incidentally, as with the general field of geriatrics, medical students receive very little education on nutrition. Although in some U.S. medical schools this subject is now a *requirement*, it is still offered by most only as an *elective*.)

This leads us now to take a look at how a variety of medications taken by older people can affect their nutritional status. Surely the physician will be careful in evaluating your parent's drug intake in this light. Does she take laxatives, diuretics, antacids, anti-convulsants, for example? Older people are particularly at risk to the effects of drugs, for certain ones can interfere with the utilization of nutrients in several ways—perhaps causing nausea, irritation of the intestinal tract, alteration of the body's sodium and potassium balance; increasing or depressing the appetite; or interfering with other bodily processes. Conversely, food can alter the rate at which needed drugs are absorbed in the body. And so, with your mother here in residence, these are important matters to be considered and explained to you by her doctor.*

Unfortunately, as we have noted, doctors themselves suffer deficient education in both nutrition and geriatrics, but there are increasing signs that medical schools are stepping up their attention to nutrition and its effect on the lifespan. Important studies remain to be carried out; soon, perhaps, scientific investigations will move to increase our knowledge.

And so, when you ask what would be a good diet for an older person, I like to quote Dr. Ruth Weg, of the Andrus

---

*For more information, write to the Drug Information Center, University of Oregon, Eugene, Oregon.

Gerontology Center, at the University of Southern California. In her book *Nutrition and the Later Years,* she reminds us that "general concepts in relation to food at any age relate as well to older persons." And she wisely notes that nutrition is more than food. She sees motivation toward eating, cultural attitudes and practices, general mental and physical health, companionship versus isolation, availability of food, geography, transportation, economics, and education as all being significant factors in the use of food. All these aspects contribute to the eating habits of any given individual. We should certainly consider this total picture of nutrition if faced with nutritional inadequacies in any specific nursing home—not an unlikely possibility, since such inadequacies have long been recognized as a priority problem in institutions for the aged.

Here we must pose another question: Are laxatives a part of Mother's care plan? Are they used sparingly, or is their routine use accepted without question? Are laxatives the easy answer to bulk deficiencies in diet and to lack of exercise?

Where, when, and how easily does your mother eat? The "how" refers to dentures. Are they loose-fitting, unused, or otherwise contributing to poor eating habits of your parent—even, in extreme cases, to malnutrition? Is staff careful in the care of dentures or tooth-brushing on a regular basis? Or can Mother do this for herself?

Focusing on food, we have checked out the meals, the kitchen, the personnel in charge, and their philosophy toward this component of holistic care. Yes, meals should be the highlight of Mother's day, the spark to enhance her other activities. For, as Virginia Woolf observed, "One cannot think well, love well, sleep well if one has not dined well."

When Mother enters the dining room, if that is where she eats, may she, too, with a shine in her eyes, delight in that welcome announcement, "Dinner is served!"

The above are some of the therapies offered in some of our geriatric homes. And may I say, probably concurring with your sentiments, that when nursing homes hire more therapists;

when doctors, rather than shrugging off a patient with "Just keep him comfortable," begin to grasp the vast potential for *creative* geriatric practice; when they write orders for therapy for *every* person in that home (including the dying, utilizing the Hospice concept); when staff envisions the highest potential and capabilities of their individual charges—only then can we claim that the American nursing home "has arrived." It will then have approached more nearly the ideal of the Scandanavian or the Soviet Union geriatric facility—or, what the Chinese call their "House of Respect." (They also call it the "Happy Home.")

In many European countries dramatic improvements in patients are seen where therapy is built into the woodwork, so to speak. Residents tend their own gardens; they create exquisite salable items, such as slippers and eyeglass cases, and for their work they are paid wages. All residents join in daily exercise, mild or strenuous. Some even jog.

The U.S. nursing facility has yet to learn the real meaning of *rehabilitation*. Most offer to a *few* residents *some* of the therapies and activities discussed in this chapter. But we look to the nursing home of the future as a vitally alive "Center for Living"—weekends as well as weekdays.

Let's get rehabilitation on the road. Cling to the belief that, to a large degree, the physical and mental ailments of the elderly are preventable and, frequently, reversible. Help these people to help themselves. "Give a man a fish," says the Chinese proverb, "and he will eat for a day. Teach him to fish and he eats for a lifetime." Therein lies our belief in therapy—for full human dignity.

Think therapy. But not just for the chosen few. Think therapy for your parent and for every living soul in that nursing home.

Parents' age must be remembered both for joy and for anxiety.
Confucius

8
When Mother Is "Difficult"

Does your parent frequently become angry? Or act helpless? Does she deny reality? Or complain constantly? Make unreasonable demands? Refuse to cooperate? Given her unique personality, plus various reasons for these kinds of behaviors, we can offer here only a few tip-of-the-iceberg suggestions. We need to be aware of these problems in geriatric facilities and to seek ever-more-satisfying solutions.

To start with, Mother herself is not "difficult"; it is her behavior which is sometimes difficult. Generally, when a person has a problem, she has a need to communicate it to others, especially if she has a hearing or sight loss. Perhaps, unable to explain her concern, she feels misunderstood, neglected, taken for granted, abused or feels the loss of control over her life. Sooner or later, like the volcano, these feelings will erupt, gently or violently.

Feelings? That's what we're talking about. Feelings, remember, are always valid, whether positive or negative. There is no such thing as a wrong feeling, an unworthy feeling. And you cannot eradicate feelings by scolding, punishing, shaming, or sedation—certainly not by announcing, "It's all in your head!" or "There, now, no sense in giving up or being upset!"

Barring a psychotic condition requiring psychiatric consultation, one helpful approach to any negative behavior might be: "Thanks, Mother, for sharing your feelings with me. Given your situation, I can understand how you feel. Can we work this out together, or to whom should we talk about them?" (Clergy, social worker, head nurse, mental health worker?)

Let's take a closer look at some of these feelings and behaviors.

Anger: Is Mother able to communicate her real feelings without fear of reprisal in the home? Anger, suppressed, can result in depression. Ventilated, it can have certain positive functions, such as unbottling hostility that otherwise might be turned inward. Anger is understandable for the chronically ill person who is confined; that patient needs constructive outlets for this emotion. But how can it be handled creatively? Perhaps the way they did it with Mrs. Finnegan?

Tillie Finnegan—a veritable battle-axe! Hell hath no fury like this woman! She delighted in kicking people in the shins, cussing them out. Ignoring her had never worked. So one day we tried a new tactic. Approaching her, I ventured a cheery "hello." But I came too close. "Don't you 'hello' me, you rotten old so-and-so," she retorted, swinging her fist and bruising my arm. But I fooled her. "Why Tillie," I exclaimed, "you must be Irish! I just love that old Irish spirit in you—what spunk, what sparkle in those blue eyes when you flash your hash like that! You *are* Irish, aren't you?"

Pulling back in utter disbelief at my reaction, she began to thaw. Then she proudly proceeded to brag of her Dublin ancestry. For the first time she told me of her frustration with her inability to walk. Her temper gradually diminished. She became the "darling" of the home. Everyone adored her flashing eyes and her wit. She allowed me to give her walking lessons.

That marvelous energy was channeled into constructive activities.*

Anger? What had we done? First of all, in a nonjudgmental way, we had validated or acknowledged her feelings. Then we had conveyed our own concern, had focused on her abilities rather than disabilities, and had upheld her dignity.

Helplessness: The next concern you may encounter in your parent is helplessness. Is this something new since she came to the home, or has she always exhibited this behavior? Unwilling to lift a finger? Ask yourself, Why does she seem to prefer helplessness to independence? What message is she trying to convey? or have we unwittingly closed the path to her independence, perhaps because of our own need to nurture or because it seems more convenient?

Look around any geriatric facility. See those mother-smotherers who are gushing over their parent like geysers? See that Mr. Bell over there—he's abdicated from life. His overly solicitous family had made him quit thinking, quit doing for himself. Although he was eventually rehabilitated and sent home, it wasn't long before his family had resmothered him right back into the nursing home.

Catering—overnursing—may be quicker and easier, but what misguided kindness—to do for a person when he can, or could, learn to do for himself! And how about that blind lady over there? A busy nurse is trying to feed her but jabs her in the cheek with a spoonful of oatmeal. "What's this?" cries the patient, when she is told that she has to be fed. "Give me that spoon," she cries, "I can do it myself"—and she proceeds to demonstrate. "After all," she mutters, "*I* know where my mouth is!"

Then there was Belle, who, after her husband's stroke, refused to smother him. Whenever they rode the elevator, for

---

*Adapted from chapter 1, "Making Geriatric Nursing Creative," in *How to Put JOY into Geriatric Care*, 2nd enlarged ed. (Bend, OR: Geriatric Press, 1979), by Nancy Littell Fox.

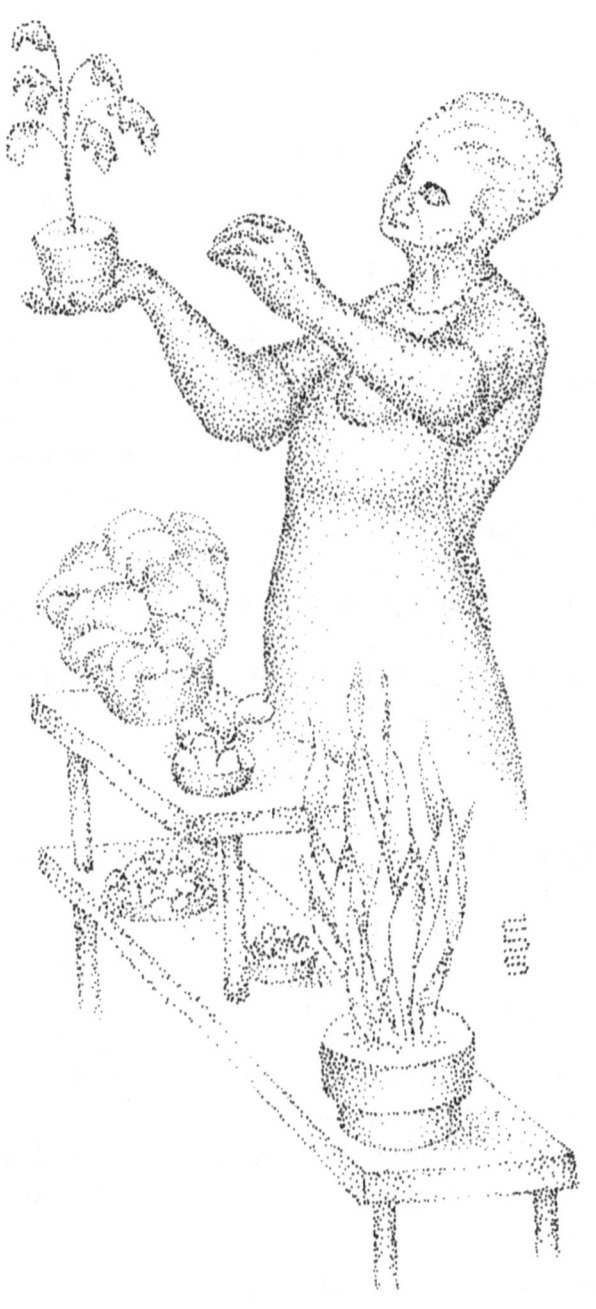

"I was becoming discontented and I found peace in tending my window-garden."

example, she insisted that Ted press the appropriate button. In his confusion, he would often press the wrong one so that up and down, down and up they would ride. My, what a lot of time they spent in that machine! But Ted finally mastered the task. In refusing to smother him, Belle won that round. But Ted was the real winner.

We used to think that a patient such as Mr. Hardy, the "exhibitionist," was "just looking for attention." And then we realized—sure, he is looking for attention because he *needs* attention! Lonely, starved for praise and encouragement, for recognition of himself as a man of dignity and worth, he indulged in bizarre behavior to gain attention. Once the staff realized this, they gave him double, triple the attention and took an interest in him as a person. Soon his behavior changed. Mr. Hardy became more self-sufficient. He even helped around the home by watering plants and pushing wheelchairs. Chapter 10, "For Your Parent, Life More Abundant," will offer some ideas about how your "helpless" parent may find greater independence.

Denial of Reality: Another negative behavior, *denial,* is well-known to health care personnel and to relatives. "Nothing's wrong with me," says Mother, "I'm fine—everything's coming up roses!" Yet, each time you visit, you note that woebegone look on her face. Could it be that the burden is too great for her to face the reality of her condition? That she does not really understand her physical condition and prognosis? Perhaps this unrealistic dreaming is her way of staying afloat. Setting up defenses is a common way of coping, yet it is hard for the relative to understand a parent who bluffs like the lady in the commercial:

Husband: How are you feeling today?
Wife: Fine and dandy, Dear. Just fine! [*But mutters under her breath:* "Darn this arthritis; it's killing me!"]

Try to bulldoze Mother into admitting a problem, and she may deny it all the more, may develop greater anxiety. Tread softly. This way you may help her take a more realistic view. She may then become more receptive to therapy and rehabilitation.

Incessant Demands: Is Mother forever complaining, demanding? I doubt that if I were chronically ill myself, I could be chronically charming when (a) the staff is too rushed to notice me, (b) I'm lonely and scared, and (c) I feel my independence slipping down the drain.

In the first place, find out if Mother's complaints are legitimate. (See discussion of grievances in chapter 11, pages 150-156.) If not, does she complain about trivia, covering up what is *really* bothering her? "I dislike the desserts here," she may say, when she means, "I can't stand the attitude of that head nurse." What is the message behind her complaints? Is she concerned about her health, her future? Then, could she be given more responsibility for her own care, more information about her own care-plan and about the goals set for her? Has she enough to do to keep mind, body, and spirit active—things to do both for herself and for others? Both short- and long-term projects? Does she feel needed? Is her advice sought? Is she still a part of your family in her own mind? Does she belong to the Resident Council? Is she a Resident Volunteer?* If these suggestions are within her capabilities and are offered to her, Mother will be too busy to complain.

Yes, Mother, herself, is never difficult. It is her behavior which can be difficult. The wonder of it all is the ability of older people to cope. They can be valiant and courageous; and they have shown these traits in the face of momentous changes in their lifestyles. Think of it—the world-shaking changes they have seen from the horse-and-buggy days to the space age!

Mother *had* to be hardy to have survived all that! Plus the losses. Her spouse, perhaps? Hearth and home, friends and

---

*In some homes, a handsome lapel pin which says *Resident Volunteer* is provided for those who wish to help push wheelchairs, feed the bedridden, greet guests, check outside for litter, and so on. Thus their renewed feeling of usefulness and dignity is enhanced.

loved ones—lost perhaps through death or relocation, social changes, financial status. A marvel, these aged ones. And the miracle? That more are not angry, rebellious, demanding, uncooperative, complaining, or generally "difficult." Truly a valiant, a grand generation!

It is worthy of note that a recent report by researchers, Drs. Costa and McCrae at the National Institute on Aging's Gerontology Research Center in Baltimore, Maryland, concludes that (a) it is not true that older people worry and complain excessively about their health and (b) the proportion of hypochondriacs among the elderly is no higher than among other age groups.

When Mother is "difficult," then, help her work out her feelings. Remember, complaints are probably not directed at you, personally. See them as her cry for help, as manifestations of inner turmoil due, most likely, to her many losses. Validate her feelings. She knows you care, but let her know you understand, that you will work with her and staff to eradicate the causes of discontent.

So Mama sometimes kicks up her heels and becomes obnoxious—causing you to feel apologetic, embarrassed? Would you want her always to conform to the sometimes deadly rules of congregate living—to be forever "manageable," docile, obedient, sticky-sweet? Or could it be that she is showing a bit of spunk and independence? Hear what she may be saying: "I'm still somebody, and if necessary, I'll stand on my head to prove it. I'm still around. And don't you forget it!"

We cease loving ourselves if no one loves us.
Madame de Stael

9
Sexuality at Any Age: Part of Being Human

Before we talk about sexuality and the aging—and why this concerns relatives of the nursing-home client—let me share with you a story, "To Have and To Hold," about a couple in a home.

"I take thee to be my (wife) (husband) to have and to hold from this day forward, for better or worse, for richer or poorer, in sickness and in health, to love and to cherish, until death us do part."

It was their fiftieth wedding anniversary. In a little ceremony in the nursing home, Ralph and Amy repeated their marriage vows, reliving that happy day so long ago. Golden daffodils, yellow roses, and candles adorned the lace-covered table. And now, Ralph was cutting the yellow-frosted cake—a gift from the nursing home. From the record player floated the soft strains of "O Promise Me."

Amy was teary-eyed. Ralph, too, was visibly overcome by the flow of loving attention from staff, family, and friends. Even Mr. Case, the administrator, was there, cordially shaking every hand.

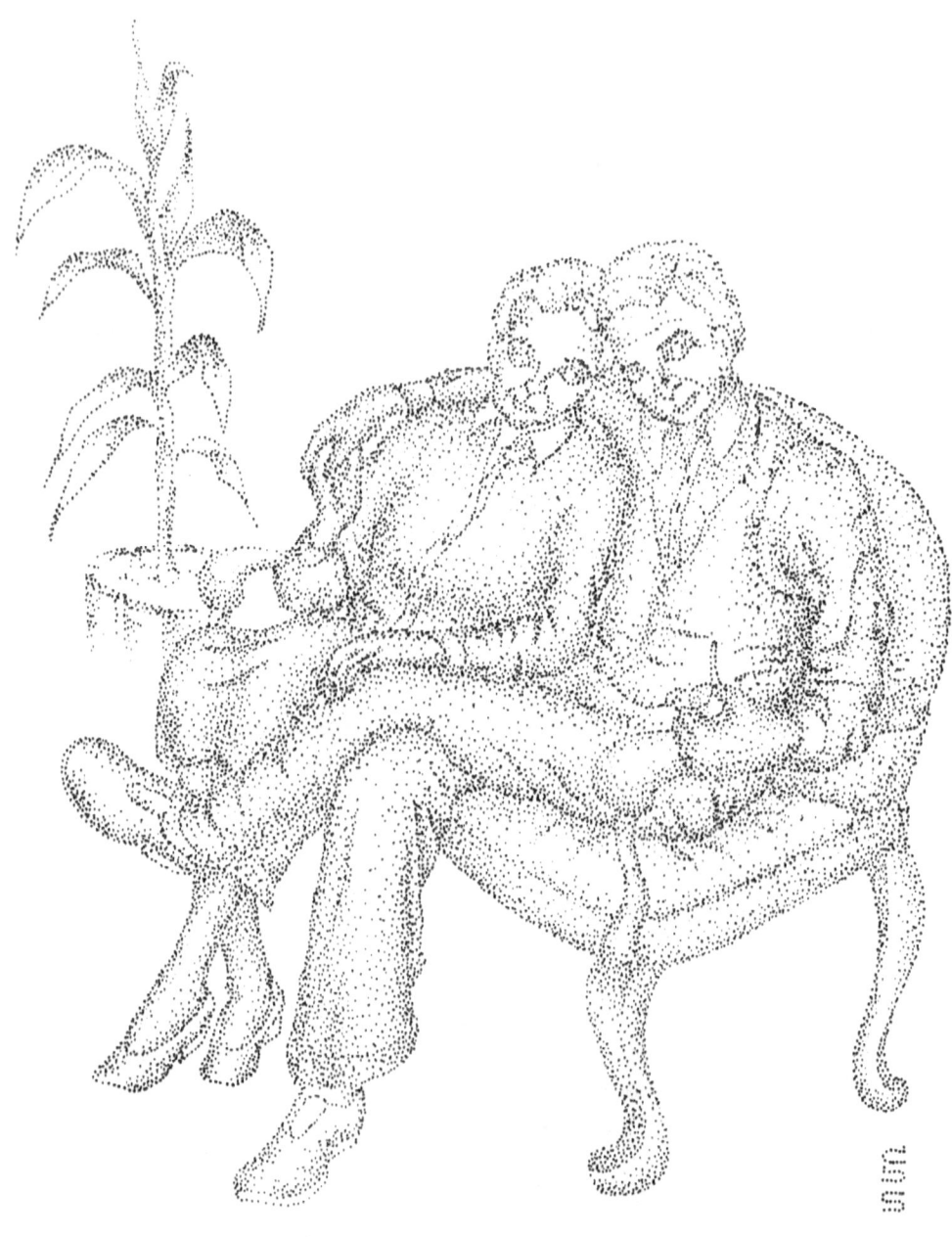

"We met in the nursing home. Both of us had lost our partners. We fell in love. We were married here. We share a room. We have our privacy. We are happy."

And then it was all over. The guests departed. Again, all was quiet. Ralph put his arms around his wife and kissed her. Nurse Nora wheeled him back to his room. Then, with assistance, Amy walked back to her room, where her bedridden roommate, Mrs. Dobbins, waited to hear all about it.

"To have and to hold"? "Until death us do part"? That night as she lay in bed, the phrases kept ringing in Amy's head. And other words kept resounding in Ralph's mind—"Those whom God hath joined together. . . ." He sighed. "Why may not Amy and I stay together, nights as well as days?" he wondered.

All of their married life, in sickness and in health, Ralph and Amy had shared a room and shared a bed. But now, in the still of the night, there was no way to lie beside her or to put his arms around her—tonight of all nights—to remind her again what a beautiful life-partner she was and always had been. Never again would they feel the closeness and warmth of one another, nor, with a soft embrace, express their need, their love—never again to have and to hold.

Must they live out their ebbing lives in separation? There remained so little time. But here in an institution, who would understand? Who would know what they meant to one another or what feelings they concealed in their hearts?

That evening, as Mr. Case was driving home, he also relived the joyous occasion. And he, too, turned over in his mind certain phrases—perhaps recalling his own marriage vows: "In sickness and in health," "A comfort in sorrow, a companion in joy," "Let no one put asunder."

On the next afternoon, Nurse Nora wheeled Ralph, as usual to visit his wife in her room. But today, something was different. The bed next to Amy's was vacant. Photos, clothes—everything had been removed from that area. Mrs. Dobbins had consented to move in with another friend.

"That bed—it's for *you!*" smiled Nurse Nora. "Mr. Case thought you might like this new arrangement. . . ."

. . . from this day forward!

Throughout their married life, your parents, too, shared "bed and board." They, too, like Ralph and Amy, may have suffered many a heart-wrench—loss of job, separation from family and friends, family tragedies. The hurt, the memory of these events are deeply inscribed in the hearts of older people, especially as they experience the trauma, as many do, of entering an institution. And so, wherever possible, couples need to room together, when this is their desire. Affection, togetherness, the expression of love in all its manifestations—should not these be encouraged by every possible means?

"We all need love," says the cliché, But do we really mean *all*? Even nursing-home residents? Even your aging parent or parents? And even if this love includes sexual expression?

It is hard for you, yes, almost impossible for us members of younger generations to imagine, let alone admit, that aging, widowed Victorians might now be attracted to one another; might experience stirrings of desire. Perish the thought!

Whence, then, cometh the phrase, "Dirty old man"? The young aide doesn't emit that howl, does she, because old Milton merely smiled at her? At his age could he possibly—yes, he just possibly . . . !

With your parent now participating in congregate living, you may want to confront this subject of sexuality among the aging—a topic you must have wondered about, and one which, for too long, has been ignored or mishandled by staff and relatives alike.

From birth to retirement, most people stay close to family, friends, and spouse. But in that last cycle of life, when the need to belong intensifies, yet another heartbreak may come. Some needs are unmet. Should the older person so much as hint he's even heard of sex—whoa! Quick, the tranquilizer!

Still, from crib to casket, love and sex are on our minds. Your mind. Mine. Everybody's mind. For, as the vine needs sunlight, so, at any age, human beings need warmth, closeness, nurturing, cherishing. Withhold this and, like bread from a toaster, up pops a problem, perhaps sickness, real or imagined. Well or ill, there is no question—sexuality is part of being human; and our humanness is part of each of us, at any age. Based on current data, it is normal for the long-lived person to have sexual feelings and fantasies, a means of acting-out behavior. What happens if these are denied?

First, what do we mean by "sexuality"?

The word "sexuality" contains five syllables. Sex is only one of them. The full meaning of sexuality might be seen as that spark within us that validates our wholeness, our integrity, our innate worth. It is the acceptance of self, in the knowledge, as the Psalmist puts it, that "we are fearfully and wonderfully made." And so, sexuality, at any age, is our bridge to human relating. And think—isn't it only through the senses that people can cross that bridge?

What if the senses are impaired? What if this bridge to communication is crumbling through failing sight and hearing, through loss of speech? There is one great consolation. Touch. Perhaps for some, touch is the only sense that lasts a lifetime. No wonder that old man or woman reaches out, grabs you as you pass by.

Aware of the implications of sensory loss, then, can we acknowledge the older person's need for closeness and human relating? The administrator of a 700-bed facility once boasted to me: "Here all the residents' needs are taken care of!" And yet, half of those people appeared drugged. In the light of today's gerontological research, are we so sure that sedation can substitute for loving, for full living? Are we so sure that it takes care of all needs? Or merely staff needs? Forcing residents into an asexual vacuum seems strange therapy to relieve feelings of isolation.

In his "Hierarchy of Needs," Abraham Maslow* rates "love needs" only one ladder-rung behind basic food and safety requirements.

---

*The late psychologist, Brandeis University.

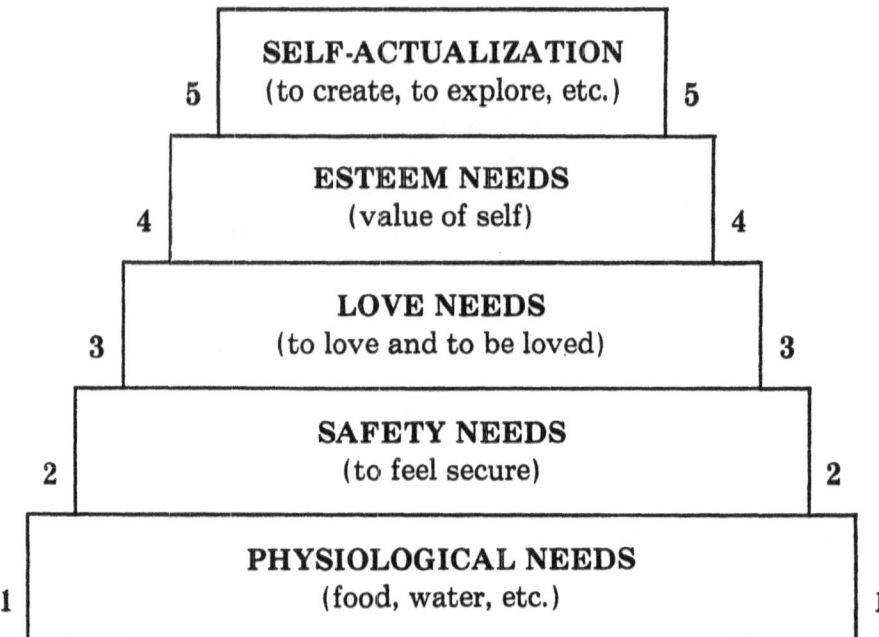

What are these love needs we're talking about? Says Dr. Lester Kirchendall, gerontologist and sex specialist, "Human relating begins with the following seven conditions: Confidentiality, trust, empathy, affectional expression, emotional investment, mutuality of motivation, and sexual expression." When two people share these values, when we acknowledge their need for freedom of expression within the bounds of privacy and good taste, are we not contributing to the dignity, self-esteem, and well-being of that couple? No longer can we assume that simply because of an accumulation of years, nursing home residents are content to sit snugly in a state of sexless senility.

You, the relative, can jolt people from believing such concepts. For, despite the persistence of societal myths concerning the aged, you probably know that aging, itself, does not cause cessation of that normal physiological function, that is, the sexual response. Perhaps you are also aware of scientific studies which tell us that a woman's libido, barring certain kinds of illness, can last a lifetime, and that the male, despite a gradual decline, can sustain desire and performance into his nineties and beyond.

Supporting this, surveys by Dr. Alexander Leaf, Massachusetts General Hospital, show that in Pakistan, Equador, and the Soviet Caucasus, large numbers of centenarians work hard, never retire, are highly respected, and remain sexually active. Further, Duke University studies show that 70 percent of males aged sixty-eight are sexually active. Masters and Johnson findings also indicate sustained interest, desire, and performance in late years. And yet, our society clings to the myth that older people simply shift into neuter. We continue to struggle with Victorian fallout—that tragic denial of sexuality in the older person. Opening our minds and hearts, may we become ever more sensitive to the deeper needs of the older generation. For, as biologist-gerontologist Alexander Comfort bluntly states: "Patients don't forfeit their civil rights by having reached a certain chronological age. Nursing homes, rehabilitation centers, and even acute hospitals will have to change their attitudes about sex among patients. I think it would be possible," he says, "to sue a nursing home for compromising patients' rights and I hope somebody does it!"

We do not advocate inappropriate behavior in institutions. We do need, however, to analyze the role we play as staff and relatives and friends. Difficult as it is to formulate, what is *your* philosophy regarding sexuality and aging, in general? And if your widowed mother develops a new love interest, can you accept this? Can you be thankful for her happiness? Will you understand that this in no way minimizes the love she will always hold for your father? Mother has so little time left. She has been lonely.

Let's talk now of late-life marriage. It could happen to your parent. It could even happen, in time, to you.

Marriage exists for the fulfillment of each partner as an entity and for the couple as a team. The young have no monopoly on marriage. And yet, what killjoys our older lovers encounter when an unsympathetic relative, now in a position of authority, objects to their union! If you were to say, "But I just can't imagine Mother . . ." or "There are too many legal tangles . . .," one could see your point of view; for truly, there have been formidable obstacles, economic and cultural, to late-life marriage. But consider. With professional advice, together with your loving support, could these tangles be unraveled? Perhaps, after all, you *could* imagine your widowed mother, if she wants it, radiant in a new love relationship. A pity her chances are slim. In the nursing home, women outnumber the men at least three to one.

Weddings do take place in nursing homes. I attended one ceremony by the bedside of the paralyzed groom. Sitting by, in her wheelchair, the beautiful, flower-bedecked eighty-three-year-old bride joined in repeating the vows. Lighted candles. A smiling staff as witness. Such joy! and for eleven months, this couple shared six out of the seven "conditions for human relating," as explained by Dr. Kirchendall. The final cycle of their lives had been enriched.

In her *Album of People Growing Old,* Shura Saul tells of an institutionalized couple who fell in love. With renewed *joie de vivre* and determination, they were able to leave the nursing home and for three years, with the help of visiting nurses and homemakers' services, shared an apartment. This had been arranged with the blessing of the wise administrator and family of the couple. Then, no longer able to cope, they returned as planned to the nursing home. What if they had been denied those three years of special togetherness?

In the home where your mother resides, what is the administration's philosophy regarding sexuality? Does it provide double rooms for couples, double beds for those who want them, as spelled out in the patients' bill of rights? What about privacy? Is there a difference between the beliefs of the staff and what it feels it must do to maintain the "image" of the home?

A theologian once said, "Love is that approach which brings to a person and to his/her situation the greatest benefit of good." For Mother, of course, you seek the "greatest benefit" according to her situation. As her adult child, you wish her joy up to the very last moment of her life. You wish her freedom of expression and control over her own affairs to the greatest extent possible. Above all, you wish her love.

May all of us, relatives and friends, afford our parents the humanizing experience of beauty and love—enabling them to grow in their humanity!

Come to think of it, is the sunset any less beautiful than the sunrise?

To finish the moment, to find the journey's end in every step of the road, to live the greatest number of hours, is wisdom.

Ralph Waldo Emerson

10
For Your Parent, Life More Abundant

Kith and kin, you cannot do it all—can't be with your mother *all* the time. You have other family and community commitments. Yet, haunted by thoughts of her unmet needs, you tossed restlessly last night, recalling recent visits to the home. Several times you found that there had been no nursing assistant to walk Mother—doctor's order says "twice a day." Especially weekends, you find her parked in that vacant lot, the corridor, along with the rest of the wheelchair brigade—no meters to indicate that her time there has expired, not even a cop to ticket her vehicle for overtime violation. Gazing mindlessly at the wall, she hardly notices the plaque admonishing her, in words attributed to St. Francis, to "accept that which you cannot change." Oh, how the hours drag!

Even though she finds some relief during occasional encounters with the therapist, even when you find her in company with others at a social program, you sense her loneliness. And especially disturbing are those times when you sense her awareness of the tedium of the TV set—rarely in focus, blaring noisily, seemingly attempting to blot out the emptiness and silence of the hours. What does Mother care about that violent shoot-out, that wrestling match where bodies are pounded to a pulp, that catfood commercial? Resigned to their fate, residents, like robots, are sometimes plunked before television, expected to be grateful, as is the itinerant preacher, "for all God's mercies."

Family is busy. Staff is overwhelmed. Weekend staff is gone with the wind.* How, then, can more spark, color, and life be added to enrich these dreary hours?

Let me tell you of a volunteer group that is tackling the problem. I believe this chapter is important even though you, as a relative, may not have the time just now to participate in such a group. But you are in a position to "talk it up" to your club or church. This group is making a difference, revitalizing minds and bodies of the confined elderly. It brings life more abundant, a closer bond between nursing homes and the community. We think it is exciting, with ever increasing potential for further benefits.

What is this group and how does it work?

Our "Ministry with Aging" project, based in Bend, Oregon, is a group from Trinity Episcopal Church which is dedicated to the proposition that *there is no such thing as a good nursing home that is not backed by the strong winds of community support.* The *immediate* goal? To broaden the horizons of the institutionalized elderly while broadening our own. The *long-term* goal? To "cover the waterfront," so that every one, of the estimated 50 percent in institutions who receives no visitors, can have a friend. The overall aim is to open up paths, to fling wide the gates, to accelerate a national trend to make nursing homes and related facilities *Centers for Living,* easily accessible to communities, schools, clubs, churches; to make them places

---

*Except for those few facilities where staff operates on a 4-2-4-2 basis (four days on duty, two days off, etc.). A model for this plan, working successfully, can be found at the Byron Health Care Center in Fort Wayne, Indiana.

for sharing, working, creating, enjoying together—all benefiting and learning, one from another. The Oregon project has a four-point plan:

- The one-to-one concept
- Love-and-learn meetings
- Mix and Match
- The Backup

Step One: Remember the Frank Laubach motto for combating world illiteracy: "Each One Teach One"? Our motto says: "Each One Adopt One." One volunteer for one resident. Why the stress on one-to-one? Look at our mental institutions, filled with people who have never known a close confidant. As the song goes: "Everybody Needs a Certain Someone."

Step Two: Meetings? Yes, but not simply coffee-klatches. Monthly Learning Opportunities. Pleasant get-togethers to prepare the volunteer for the task. (What job in this world can you think of that does not require systematic preparation, orientation, ongoing continuing education?) Through discussion, reading aloud together, films, slides, and invited speakers, volunteers become excited about improving skills, stretching personal horizons.

Meetings are unstructured, geared to the questions in our minds. Right now we are studying the therapeutic value of reminiscence. We have worked on the therapeutic value of poetry for older persons as well as the value of pets, music, singing, and praying. We have studied some particular situations such as communicating with older people who have vision or hearing impairments. We are now working with a speaker who is donating her time to bring about a better awareness of the needs of the terminal patient—to make dying "an act worth doing well," as author Arthur Gordon puts it. This is a group of people learning and growing together, people with a purpose, who, in giving of themselves and their time, show tangible benefits for both volunteer and resident.

For Your Parent, Life More Abundant / 137

Step Three: Mix-and-Match is another part of the program that is sheer fun. The new volunteer makes an appointment to see the head nurse or activities director, who asks about the volunteer's interests and background. And while the volunteer talks, can't you see the head nurse say to herself: "Aha! Won't this person be *per*fect for old Mrs. Grady in Room 69, who *also* adores caterpillars, cauliflower, and Kansas!" You won't be matched with a deaf person if you yourself are hard-of-hearing! Mix and match? For compatible relationships, it's almost a no-fail recipe!

Step Four: The Backup System. Suppose the volunteer is ill, out of town, or tied up with a croupy husband. Will her adoptee be disappointed, wait in vain for that weekly visit? Enter now the Backup. This is the friend invited to be a stand-in when needed. The Backup is introduced to Mrs. Grady *before* her first visit, so that she already knows the resident's preferences—her fondness for backrubs, apple-strudel, and country rides. And so, as we watched, the Ministry with Aging, like Topsy, "growed."

Starting with two members, we now have eighteen who have shown their interest. Eighteen people to befriend eighteen residents of nursing homes. We hope it will grow until *every* lonely resident has his or her friendly visitor. Our system works because that backup person, once she visits, finds it fulfilling. She now wants an adoptee for herself, asks to join our group. "Not yet!" we tell her. First you need to attend two of our meetings and become familiar with the four-point process. You, too, must be mixed and matched with the right person for you.

Through this system, people learn how involvement, which can be as limited as a person wants it to be, can be deeply satisfying. It is an answer to the person who longs to help but says: "That's not my thing" or "I hate to visit a nursing home—it's so depressing!"

Depressing? No longer true of many of them, for our society is requiring changes. Let your light so shine that *you* set the tone: *you* turn apathy into aliveness in the nursing facility, *you* transform visitations from dormant, nonevents to active, creative happenings. Because of you, the volunteer, one older person can look forward to each new day.

"Can a volunteer be liable, or sued?" you ask. What if, even with a signed permission slip to leave the premises, an accident occurs when I take a resident for an outing? My attorney tells me no, "not unless gross negligence can be proved." (That is, if you are not performing a paid service.)

What kind of volunteer is needed? Spare the facility that goody-goody semi-annual drop-in—you know, the one who, to ease conscience, sashays down the hall, waves at residents, bedecks the nursing station with garish gladioli, then disappears. Such a person is not ready for serious volunteering. But don't discount her—she may be recruitable!

Relatives, tell your friends. Tell your neighbors enthusiastically about the project. Help to get it started in your town, or amalgamate with a local volunteer group. Demonstrate the joy of adopting one of the older generation; show your friends how, through a learning-and-love-directed ministry, they can respark a life. In the process, they will discover that it matters not one whit what a person does, earns, or owns; that in the eternal scheme of things, it matters only who he is. For each volunteer and adoptee there awaits something wonderful—life more abundant!

The objective of this ministry is to combat loneliness in the institution. With a similar objective in mind, Duane Valentry wrote the following article which is filled with good ideas for the volunteer.

When you have said "hello" to your adoptee and covered the pleasantries, what next? Valentry will tell you:

Leave the Flowers Home*

Anyone who has spent time in a hospital or nursing home contemplating the shadows on the wall, knows how

---
*Reprinted by special permission of *The Rotarian*, December, 1975.

the hours creep by. "Intense boredom affects about ten percent of our population, including the aged, and many who are institutionalized," says Dr. Mark, of the U.S. Department of Health. "Anyone who sits around and does nothing all day gets badly depressed. Sooner or later, some will have suicidal thoughts."

To combat institutional boredom, Dr. Mark has developed an ingenious idea called "Prev**lab**" (preventing **l**oneliness, **a**nxiety, and **b**oredom). The Prevlab theory is simple: Give the confined individual something to divert him—stimulate his mind.

Dr. Mark observes that many patients have flowers and plants, but these don't occupy their thoughts, time or hands. He began taking them other presents—old magazines, menus, travel schedules, games, cartoons, clippings, and puzzles. As interest grew he became more imaginative.

"Hey, this magazine is really something!" said one patient. "I remember all these things that happened that year. I showed it to my friends, and we spent the whole afternoon looking through and discussing it."

Those words: "spent the whole afternoon" stuck in Dr. Mark's mind. The simple idea worked. Why not expand on it with multi-hobby kits for these lonely people?

It didn't take much time or money to make up a kit—just caring and imagination. He tucked in items he found on walks through the woods and parks: stones, leaves, driftwood, dried flowers. The results were marvelous! An elderly woman, victim of an auto crash, was often in tears from sheer boredom. Dr. Mark stuffed some "things" in a basket and strolled in to see her one afternoon. The basket contained literally hundreds of items of all descriptions—catalogues, crayons, masks, games, shells, coins, etc. The patient became a new person!

It is Dr. Mark's opinion that fine new institutional facilities are great for the doctor, the technicians, the custodian, but lousy for the patient. "If I had my way," he says, "every place for the long-term care patient would be a cultural center, with alternating pictures on the wall, exhibits, lots of interesting items around, even at the risk of inviting a germ or two. A culturally sterile environment should be avoided at all times." He sees the day coming when hospital or nursing-home gift shops will stock multi-hobby kits along with flowers and useless trinkets. He offers these tips:

1) Items should appeal to the senses. They should be fun to touch or look at. They can be humorous or gimmicky, cultural or historical. They should be self-starting—not requiring prolonged or heavy concentration.

2) Items should call for active involvement or handling. They should be light-weight, inexpensive, non-perishable, pinpointed to known areas of patient interest.

3) Volunteers should mobilize community resources, calling on such groups as service clubs for suggestions, contributions, and kit assembling. Others who enjoy helping are collectors, artists, schools, drama clubs, churches.

Too many nursing homes are drab, grim places, "hardly the place a human being should spend time for improvement of physical or mental ills. Living in a nursing home should be a rich, meaningful experience."*

"Volunteers, why not check out needs of residents in local nursing homes?" asks Dr. Mark. Students, civic groups, people from all kinds of organizations can get into the act. Even pre-school children.

Look through your attic for forgotten or neglected items—an old rubber doll, a book, an old *Reader's Digest,* foreign coins, minerals, modeling clay, penny-postcards, a

---

*For vivid examples of what you can actually do (and have fun doing it), see Fox, *How to Put JOY into Geriatric Care* ($9.95 postpaid; add 18% in Canada. For address, see Appendix, p. 168).

View-Master, reels—possibilities are endless. The variety is guaranteed to give anyone on the receiving end a lot to think about besides aches and pains, hopelessness of the cracks on the ceiling and on the sterile wall.

Would that this article by Dr. Mark were available in all public libraries! It stimulated ideas from our volunteer group, such as the following:

- Read aloud or ask your adoptee to read to you. (Don't forget those large-print books at your library.)
- Maintain telephone contact with several residents.
- Encourage reminiscences. Listen actively to gain more insight into your cultural heritage. What were those days like—the politics, dress, manners, the arts, houses, etc.? Record old memories, the lore of the past, by making tapes.
- Bring babies and children for frequent visits.
- Help orient other new residents to the home—those who may have no families of their own.
- Bring in musical instruments to share or revive talents.
- How about the family pet? Ask permission to bring "it" over, or for your parent to take a walk with the pet, if possible.
- Share a glass of light wine to make a Saturday night festive, if this would bring pleasure and you have permission.
- Share yourself with a terminally ill resident. Sit with him, hold his hand, listen actively.
- Enjoy Sunday dinner with the residents (for a small fee). The home will encourage you to do this.

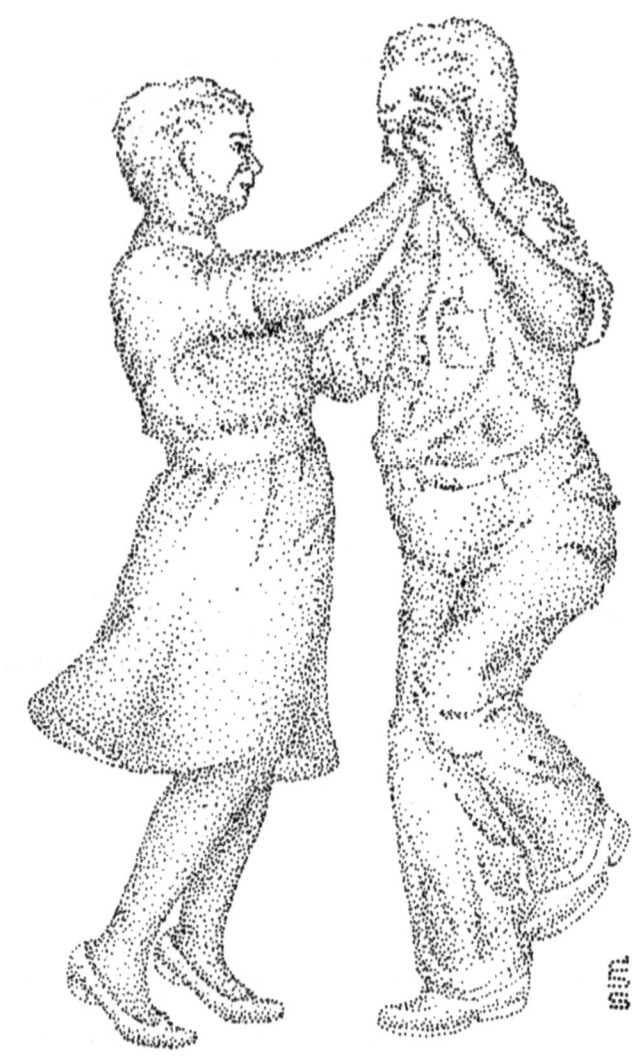

"Henry and I have always enjoyed dancing. So we were enthusiastic when weekly dances were started here."

- Ask your club to share time and talents with the residents on a regular basis. Do they sing "at," or *with,* residents? Do they make laprobes for them, or do they help the residents make them—for themselves or as gifts for others? Scrapbooks, quilts, and many other long-range projects will keep the resident looking forward to tomorrow.

- Assist with transportation to group picnics, museums, concerts, the zoo, etc., so that many more residents may be included in these outings. Or take a patient to church (you may have to sign a permission slip). How uplifting to the spirit!

- When a nursing home celebrates birthdays wholesale by the month, help a resident to celebrate retail, "by the person" on his own special day.

You and other relatives might come up with even better ideas. The Director of Volunteer Services will guide you.

Continuity-of-care is a goal of most nursing homes, meaning not just physical care. How about continuity-of-cultural-care? Is Hanukkah duly celebrated for the Jewish resident? Kosher food provided when desired? Are holidays of other countries noted, such as Bastille Day, for the resident of French ancestry? Or the Chinese New Year? Or the birthday of the English queen? For blacks and whites alike, Martin Luther King Day? And how about an Oktoberfest for the German? You can think of many others.

Be a volunteer yourself, if you can, and recruit others. Once they see the need and the void they can fill, they will rally to the task. Students, school children—all can contribute to make many lives more meaningful, more colorful.

Yes. Leave the flowers home and bring that part of you that says: "I care a whole lot." Residents have been transformed spiritually and physically when a community takes this kind of interest. It prolongs lives, the will to live. And you and your friends will be helping to fill these places with light, sounds, color, action, joy, and above all, love.

A piece of incense may be as large as the knee but, unless burnt, emits no fragrance.

Malay proverb

11
The Nursing Home Is What You Make It

Let there be no mistake! This book upholds the concept of the nursing home and stresses its value in our society for those who (1) require fulltime supervision, (2) have nowhere else to go, and (3) are forced to leave their own homes because of inadequate (or lack of) community services. We uphold the long-term care home whose adequately staffed, properly trained, respectfully salaried personnel provides quality care, whose humanitarian considerations overshadow all else.

However, we plead: Beware the facility that discovers that "there is gold in them thar wrinkles" and then capitalizes on the powerlessness of its patients. Beware the home with that windfall-profit gleam in its eye.

"But," you ask, "how can I tell one from the other? How do I tell whether the stated goals of the home tally with performance?" And the answer: Read this chapter carefully. Be aware of the six practices (outlined below), inherent in some facilities, which bear negatively on the well-being of the residents, which demonstrate that staff convenience takes precedence over patients' rights. You will not read of these in the usual How-to-Pick-a-Nursing-Home Manual, whether published by the government, the industry, or an author who has not worked in geriatric facilities. Although, in themselves, these practices (side-effects of institutionalization) are not ruinous, they depersonalize; they are bad for morale. For example, G. Janet Tulloch in her book, *A Home Is Not a Home,* refers to certain attitudes as "the eating away of self-respect and self-reliance—never an intentional act, but neither . . . intentionally prevented." Put another way (and not necessarily referring to nursing homes) Frances Storlie, R.N., observes that "cruelty can be so subtle that even the cruel don't recognize it."

1) The Float System

A nurse or nursing assistant is "floated" from floor to floor to assist wherever needed at the time.* This is a convenience for the facility that tolerates a shortage of staff but is a practice that prevents stability of environment for the geriatric resident. From one day to the next, he cannot depend upon having the same caretaker. This disorients many patients and hinders early detection of physical or mental changes. Like a bobbing lifebuoy, he is buffeted about, confused by the ever-changing faces of the staff. "And who will it be tomorrow?" he moans.

In the spring of 1980, a nursing home in Portland, Oregon, was the target of a nurses' strike whose demands included the elimination of the float system. The nurses won.

2) The Numbers Racket

In the oversized institution, your parent may overhear nurses talking. "You give Fifty-eight a bath, and I'll feed Thirty-one." It is not uncommon for a doctor to say to a nurse: "How is Forty-four today?" or, "I'll be checking out the kidney in Two-o-one."

---

*Sometimes a "float" works in this capacity *by choice.*

3) The Ping-Pong Game

Just returning from a temporary stay in the hospital, Mrs. Jones learns that, in her absence, her nursing-home bed has been reassigned. Like a ping-pong ball, she is batted around. In the "Litany of Nursing Home Abuses," the Senate Supporting Paper #1 tells how states play musical chairs with the frail elderly, moving them from room to room, floor to floor, and even from institution to institution, in whatever direction will save the most money—a practice that encourages confusion of mind. Be sure that your contract stipulates that, if hospitalized, your parent will retain her nursing-home bed, at least for a reasonable length of time.

To the patient, the shock of transplantation can be just as devastating as that experienced from "ping-ponging." Take the case of Mr. Rossi.

Although fighting like a bull, he is admitted to a facility. With no choice in the matter, no orientation, he is suddenly thrust into the shrunken environment of a cubicle—and with a disagreeable roommate, to boot. His life, he feels, has been ripped from the roots. Resentful, he withdraws, deteriorates, and joins the many who, as statistics show, do not survive their first year in a nursing home.

The shock of transplantation may greatly affect the person who is forced into entering an institution, the person who comes in kicking and screaming. It also often affects those who have been tricked into entering. An elderly person might be told, "We're taking you for a nice ride"—only to find himself deposited at the nursing home's admission office. These are the patients who, because of the thoughtless treatment and resulting shock, frequently do not survive their first year in residence.

I recall the too-sudden closing of a small, long-term-care wing of a midwestern hospital. Anxious residents wept because, for years, this had been their only home. Freighted from family, friends, and hometown, within one year, nine of the eleven residents lay in their graves.

An old man lived at the base of Mount Saint Helens. Urged

to flee as the mountain emitted volcanic ash, he bellowed: "This is my *home*! It's been my home for eighty-five years. Lava or no lava, this is where I'm staying." One month later, old Harry and his home were buried under tons of hot ash.

A Delaware facility actively works to prevent transplantation shock. Before a patient is admitted, a relative is required to bring him for two preliminary visits to meet staff and residents, to join them for at least one meal, and to spend a full weekend. Initial adjustments are softened, for the family must sign a promise to visit each day for the first two weeks (each day they must sign in) and, thereafter, once a week for as long as they live in the community. If there is no family to do this, a volunteer is enlisted to perform this service.

4) The Staff Coffee-Break

9 a.m. — this is a particular time of day when staff services are urgently needed. Yet, just about now, staff may be eying that enticing coffee-doughnut break. As the bewildered resident is whizzed through his morning ritual, staff tension increases. Even if the break is staggered, with only one employee off the floor at this time, some residents are left dangling, half-dressed, half-shaved, one sock on, one sock off. "I never eat breakfast," say many employees. *Perhaps they had better eat breakfast before they come!** Postponing the break for one hour would ease the stress all around.

5) "Mealtiming"

To what extent does the home place staff convenience above patients' rights? Take the matter of meal scheduling. Are meals served at reasonable hours and intervals? State regulations have something to say about this, but enforcement is lax. If

---

*It has been demonstrated that in industrial plants, better morale and better production is evidenced where breakfast is a requisite for employees. There are also fewer accidents on the job.

supper is served at 4:30 p.m., with a lapse of perhaps fourteen hours until the next morning's breakfast, this is a violation—unless *every* resident, with few exceptions, is offered evening nourishment. When a person awakens hungry in the middle of the night, will he be offered a glass of warm milk, perhaps, besides a comforting bedside chat and backrub? Or, will he be treated in a negative manner—as was one woman who made the request for a snack at 3 a.m. After thoroughly scolding her as if she were a child, the nurse-aide reminded her that since she had not eaten all her supper, no wonder she was hungry.

6) The Life-Care Plan

Some nursing homes offer a contract called the Life Care Contract. In exchange for a lump sum, the patient will be cared for permanently, as long as he lives. He hands over all his worldly goods, savings, investments, real estate, assets, policies. In the hands of the honest operator, this plan works well. The client feels good about not being a burden to his family. However, what happened to Mrs. Norton? In the grip of a greedy manipulator, she and her family had failed to read the contract's fine print.

Mrs. Norton had lived in the home for only six months when she developed a cold and was given extra nursing measures for her comfort. However, the administrator kept showing up in her room to see what was going on. "Don't bother," he ordered me (and the rest of the staff), "she is going to die anyway. Que sera sera!" The gleam in his eye was unmistakable. When we ignored his orders, he became angry.

When presented to relatives, the life-care plan sounds feasible. But, as the case of Mrs. Norton shows, might not an administrator build up resentment toward the life-care resident whose demise, in his opinion, is overdue? The will to live can be undermined by the unscrupulous operator for, whether the patient lives or dies, his lump sum has already been handed over. The prospect of a new windfall from a new life-care client may seem very enticing.

Ask if this home provides a probationary period of at least six months before such a contract becomes final. Will the home give a refund if your parent is not satisfied and desires a transfer? On such a transaction, be sure to consult your attorney. In some states, the home is required to hold in reserve (it can be in real estate or other equity) the same amount it has received in lump sums, so that, always, the sum can be relinquished if necessary, to the client or clients—a good safeguard for the consumer. Your attorney can check on this. The plan has proved very workable, especially in Florida.

You may now be wondering, if you detect some or all of these six practices in a facility, what you can possibly do to change, improve, or offset the effects on your parent. Linda Horn and Elma Griesel, in *Nursing Homes: A Citizens' Action Guide* (Boston: Beacon Press, 1978), state the following:

> There are forces at work in our society to promote the health and welfare of nursing home residents. Individuals, groups, organizations which are a part of that movement should be recognized and commended. As responsible citizens, we can no longer avoid our own responsibility to solve the problems inherent in the long-term-care system. Citizen involvement and community action at the local, state, and national level are necessary and vital factors for fundamental reform.

Citizen involvement and community action, then, are crucial, not only for nursing-home residents, of which there are over 1.3 million in this country, but because, as Dr. Robert Kastenbaum, of Wayne State University, observes: "While one out of twenty seniors is in a nursing home or related facility on any given day, one out of five will spend some time in a nursing home during a lifetime."

We can be certain that the nursing home of tomorrow will be exactly—no better and no worse—what we insist that it become. Like any other service, *the nursing home is what you make it.*

When You Have a Grievance

In chapter 3, "A Mighty Fortress, the Family," we emphasized the importance of making your voice heard, whether it is to praise the staff, encouraging merit and quality care, or whether it is to complain. Both approaches can be accomplished in a constructive manner. If you have a grievance, what do you do? How and to whom do you make it known?

First of all, family, look for and read the Patients' Bill of Rights. Nursing facilities are required not only to post this document in full view, but to explain it to each patient upon admission to the facility. Ask for a copy to take home with you.

The Patients' Bill of Rights is not just a listing of lofty-sounding ideals. It is the lifeline to the dignity of your mother. Not one of its stipulations should be taken lightly. Each must be fully implemented by both the institution and all visitors.

Here is the Bill. After you have read it, we will discuss the redress of grievances by means of several channels at your service.

Patients' Bill of Rights

Under Federal regulations, nursing homes must have written, updated policies covering the rights and responsibilities of patients, and these must be available to patients and to the public, to ensure that each patient in the facility:

1) Is fully informed, as evidenced by the patient's written acknowledgment, prior to, or at the time of admission and during stay, of these rights and of all rules and regulations governing patient conduct and responsibilities;

2) Is fully informed, prior to or at the time of admission and during stay, of services available in the facility, and of related charges including any charges for services not covered under title XVIII or XIX of the Social Security Act, or not covered by the facility's basic per diem rate;

3) Is fully informed, by a physician, of his medical condition unless medically contraindicated (as documented, by a physician, in his medical record), and is afforded the opportunity to participate in the planning of his medical treatment and to refuse to participate in experimental research;

4) Is transferred or discharged only for medical reasons, or for his welfare or that of other patients, or for non-payment for his stay (except as prohibited by title XVIII of the Social Security Act), and is given reasonable advance notice to ensure orderly transfer or discharge, and such actions are documented in his medical record;

5) Is encouraged and assisted, throughout his period of stay, to exercise his rights as a patient and as a citizen, and to this end may voice grievances and recommend changes in policies and services to facility staff and/or to outside representatives of his choice, free from restraint, interference, coercion, discrimination, or reprisal;

6) May manage his personal financial affairs, or is given at least a quarterly accounting of financial transactions made on his behalf should the facility accept his written delegation of this responsibility to the facility for any period of time in conformance with state law;

7) Is free from physical and mental abuse, and free from chemical and (except in emergencies) physical restraints except as authorized in writing by a physician for a specified and limited period of time, or when necessary to protect the patient from injury to himself or to others;

8) Is assured confidential treatment of his personal and medical records, and may approve or refuse their release to any individual outside the facility, except in case of his transfer to another health care institution, or as required by law or third-party payment contract;

9) Is treated with consideration, respect, and full recognization of his dignity and individuality, including privacy in treatment and in care for his personal needs;

10) Is not required to perform services for the facility that are not included for therapeutic purposes in his plan of care;

> **11)** May associate and communicate privately with persons of his choice, and send and receive his personal mail unopened, unless medically contraindicated (as documented by his physician in his medical record);
>
> **12)** May meet with, and participate in activities of social, religious, and community groups at his discretion, unless medically contraindicated (as documented by his physician in his medical record);
>
> **13)** May retain and use his personal clothing and possessions as space permits, unless to do so would infringe upon the rights of other patients, and unless medically contraindicated (as documented by his physician in his medical record);
>
> **14)** If married, is assured privacy for visits by his/her spouse; if both are in-patients in the facility, they are permitted to share a room, unless medically contraindicated (as documented by his physician in his medical record).

One wonders *why the need* to spell out a patient's bill of rights when these rights should be self-evident among any group of human beings. However, familiarize yourself thoroughly with this document which is your backbone of support if ever you have a complaint.

Have you a grievance concerning medical care—proof that proper and adequate help is not being provided? If you have approached the problem through the channels of nursing-home hierarchy with no satisfaction, and you have spoken to the doctor to no avail, you can report this professional to your county medical office or to the state licensing authority, at the Department of Health and Human Services. Ask your local health department for their address. For specific legal or ethical problems, consult your attorney or the Legal Aid Society.

What do you do for other complaints—for example, a noisy roommate who for weeks has cried out in the night, disturbing your mother's rest? What if the staff has done nothing to remedy this, although an obvious solution would be to move the roommate in with a deaf person?

As you know, good communication between you and the staff is necessary. Speak up, but speak calmly, as discussed in chapter 3, "A Mighty Fortress, the Family." Start by speaking to the direct-care aide, then to the nurse in charge and, if necessary, right up the ladder to the administrator, department of health, and area agency on aging in your state capitol—who may then contact the nursing-home ombudsman. (In many states it is the law that any abuses to patients be reported. In fact, failure to do so may bring a penalty.)

The Nursing-Home Ombudsman (or Ombudsperson)

Who and what is the nursing-home ombudsman (NHO)? This is a person who performs services at no cost to the patient. A signed letter requesting the services is all that is required. If a complainant cannot write, the ombudsman will transcribe an oral complaint and is responsible to the complainant or relatives for providing the patient with a sense of participation and self-determination, seeking to provide an effective means to ensure that he/she receives fair treatment.

The ombudsman is a public agent accountable finally to the Department of Health and Human Services and first to a wide variety of executive, administrative, and consumer agencies. The NHO is not directly accountable to the public, inasmuch as he or she is not an elected official; but he is an independent, politically neutral examiner who receives and investigates complaints from the public against nursing homes, with the power to criticize and publicize, but not to reverse any action or decision by an agency or home. An expert in nursing-home affairs, he has universal accessibility and power only to recommend. He aims to help the public—primarily patients—who question their treatment by nursing homes or nursing-home agencies. For more information, obtain the manual *Ombudsman for Nursing Homes: Structure and Process,* available from the U.S. Department of Health and Human Services, Administration on Aging publication #78-20293.

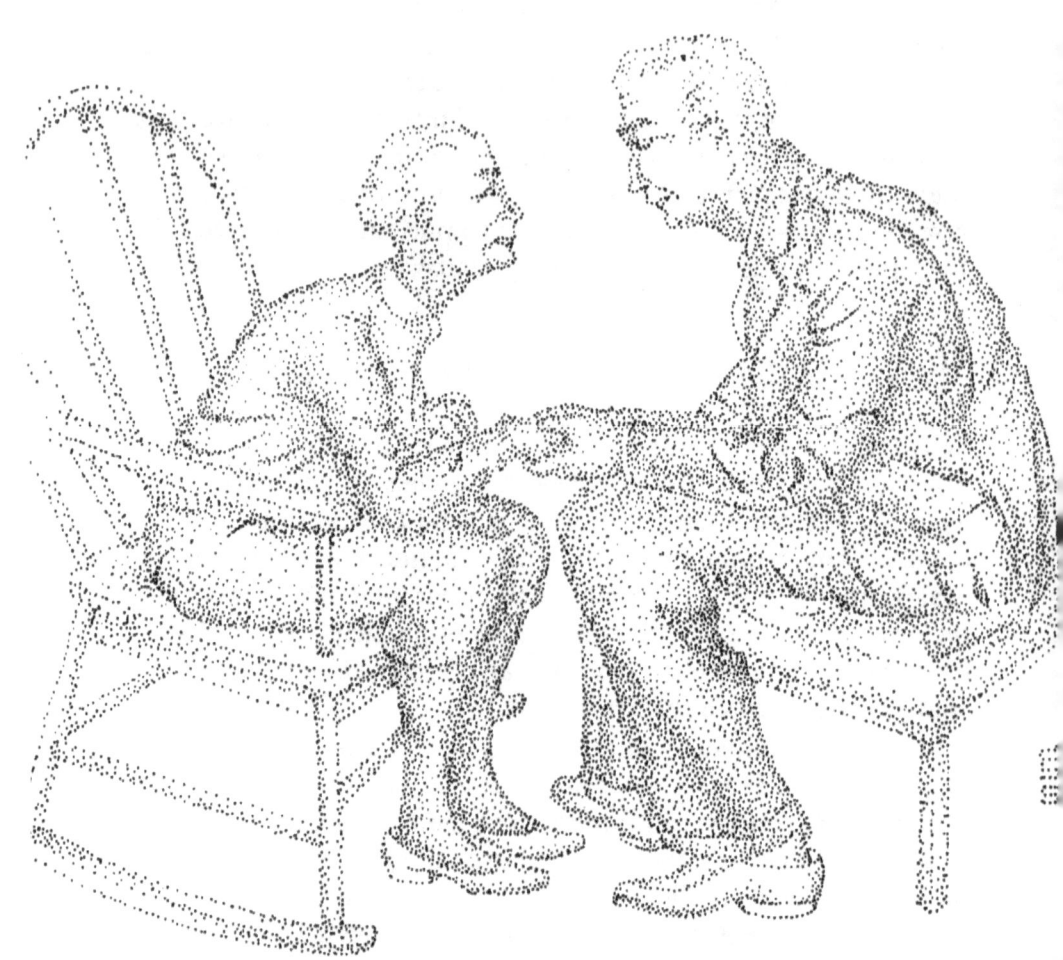

"I prefer to live in my home, but I no longer am able to. The nursing home shelters me. My family still cherishes me and I see that I keep vigorous and alert to my changing needs. I am old but my mind is still good. When I feel the need is not being met I discuss it with the staff, the director, the doctor, my spiritual counselor or I call in my family. I am lucky to have a family that is so attentive."

Grievances may also be resolved through a resident council. Many nursing homes have established this important body within the past few years. This consists of a group of residents who form a team that is the best antidote to the detrimental effects of institutional living and that serves as a stimulus for reinvolvement of the residents in the mainstream of the home and the community.

Send for the manual *How to Establish a Resident Council,* to familiarize yourself with this kind of group and what it can do for your parent. (Available from the Federation of Protestant Welfare Agencies, Division on Aging, 281 Park Avenue South, New York, NY 10010.)

You can better evaluate the attitudes of nursing-home staff and administrator if you are aware of the following common objections to organizing a resident council:

- "This home has too many old, sick, or feeble residents for us to develop a council." (This underestimates the capacity for the ailing person to participate in group discussion.)

- "As a small facility, a family-like home, we can maintain a close relationship with each and every resident—thus there is no need for a resident council." (A common argument, yet even the smallest homes have residents whose needs should be resolved democratically as a group as well as individually.)

- "Our residents are apathetic and disinterested in group activities or in starting a council." (Then something is radically wrong. Is the notion of the residents' incompetence subtly being promoted? Make a special appointment for a heart-to-heart discussion with staff. Or, a simple appraisal of behavior may reveal such attitudes. It is easier for the staff to do for the patient rather than to encourage self-help, but this promotes apathy and incompetence.*)

Gari-Lesnoff Caravaglia, Ph.D., notes, "The conscious or unconscious intentions that dominate a society are often expressed through that society's institutions." May you, the relative, be counted among those who express the intentions of your community so far as your nursing homes are concerned. The nursing home is what you make it.

> Mourn not the dead . . . mourn not your captive
>   comrade, but rather . . .
> Mourn the apathetic throng—
> The cowed and the meek—
> Who see the world's great anguish,
> And dare not speak!
>
>   Ralph Chapin

---

*How to organize, plan, and achieve nursing-home reform in your community? We recommend the book *Nursing Homes: A Citizens' Action Guide* (see Appendix).

Death is a thing of grandeur. It brings instantly into being a whole new network of relations between you and the ideas, the desires, the habits of the man now dead. It is a rearrangement of the world.

Saint-Exupéry

12
When Your Parent Is Terminally Ill

What you are going through now, others cannot know. You and your mother are unique. So is your situation. This phase of your lives is special to your whole family.

Mother lies there, her earthly journey coming to a close. You want to comfort her, but, needing comfort yourself, your emotions block the way. Even though she says, "I am ready to go when the Lord takes me," you may be devastated by the thought of ever letting her go. Or, as in some cases, a family prays that she may soon die. She has had enough. She is at the point of no return.

May I share with you something personal? It could help as, exhausted, you wait—uncertain what to do, what to say, not daring to grab an hour of sleep "just in case," and yet dreading the final moment. I hope that the insights I have gained since my own mother's death may be of value to you.

Mother died on a cold February night. I wasn't there. I did not make it from Minnesota to her nursing home in New York.

What haunts me even more is the knowledge that most people do not fear death—I'm sure she didn't—but they fear dying alone. And I, her only daughter, was not notified in time. Still, even if I *had* been there, at that stage of my life, twelve years ago, I would not have possessed the one priceless insight I can share now.

In Arthur Gordon's sensitive book *A Touch of Wonder*,* he states: "Death is not just the surrender of life, but a positive act worth doing well—an act people need help to accomplish."

Since Mother's death, during my vigils with the dying, I have thought about those words. Seen in that light, dying takes on a new dimension. No longer uncertain what to say or do during what may become a long-drawn-out process, you and your family can play an active supportive part in her passing. It can be a growing experience for both you and her. You make the act of dying creative, "a positive act worth doing well." This philosophy brings new purpose to your vigil as, over the hours, you become ever closer.

Dying, then, need not be a frightening experience. Even if it is your own mother, father, close relative, or beloved friend, you can help to make that death a victory—the serene, dignified closing of a life-cycle.

No, I was not with my mother, but there was one consolation. I was able to be with my "second mother"—my adored Aunt Alma. Let me tell what it can mean to die a "good death"—when a person is ready, when the time has come to reject "heroics" (that is, those artificial life-support measures which would only prolong her discomfort, her natural process of "moving on"). After her final, paralyzing stroke we brought Aunt Alma home. We knew she wanted to die in familiar surroundings, close to those she loved. A visiting nurse kept a check on her for, by now, her helplessness was total. No more hospital; no more subjecting her to endless tubes, needles, machines—those scientific marvels she so dreaded. No more

---
*Old Tappan, NJ: Fleming Revell, Co., 1976.

would we allow her frail body to be juggled among the staff to become everybody's—yet nobody's—patient.

In our town, "hospice" was still only a concept. And so we planned to create our own hospice to turn Aunt Alma's home into a sanctuary where she could know the love and support we had to give. As her final hours approached, rather than being wracked with torment, these hours became for us all a beautiful experience. We witnessed the gentle passing of a life to the next—to what Aunt Alma knew would be a more wonderful existence.

I don't know what you believe, nor what your parent believes. Regardless of your religious or nonreligious convictions, however, I do know this: the "creative vigil" for your mother can be a way of telling her, "I love you. I want you to know that your life has had meaning, deep meaning for me and for the family. We will always be close to you, even if you no longer dwell among us."

Here is how we spent our final hours with Aunt Alma— hours of deep significance for me, for each one of her family.*

Friday afternoon, 2:00 p.m.

Alma is comfortably settled in her own bed at home. Her temperature is rising. It is not easy to stand by and watch it spike to 103 degrees, nor to see the precipitous drop in her blood pressure. Moistening her lips and repositioning her, I stand by as she slides into an exhausted sleep. Now I recall the time she so earnestly said to me, "Nancy, in case of crisis, let me be home." It is good that she is here. She is aware.

4:00 p.m.

Aunt Alma is now awakening. Her skin is hot, but she is calm. It is good, too, that she finds emotional support in her final human experience. Her loved ones stand by, press her hand. She knows

---

*In more condensed form, this account appeared in *How to Put JOY into Geriatric Care*, by Nancy Fox.

it. I wipe her brow. She gently presses my hand, telling me what her aphasic or unspeaking sounds could never convey—that she is all right, content in the knowledge that she is dying. Her dignity and her humanness are preserved. Fortressed by a sister, a niece, and her brother, and by being here at home where she knows affection, she is being spared weeks, perhaps months, of unnecessary anguish that might have resulted from the forced lengthening of her life in the impersonal atmosphere of a hospital.

4:35 p.m.

And now, Aunt Alma, your breathing is becoming irregular. Your heart is tired, making its last effort. It would be unkind, now, if a nurse were to feel your pulse, or flaunt before you a cold stethoscope. Instead, I am putting my arm around her shoulder, holding her secure, helping to cross the threshold. It won't be long now.

5:00 p.m.

Aunt Alma, your lips and mouth are again becoming dry. It is not too late to swab them gently, one more time. Do I discern an almost imperceptible smile, as if you were trying to tell us this helps a little bit?

It may be that now Aunt Alma cannot hear well, but her sister puts a record on the player—her favorite hymns, and then, her beloved "New World Symphony." It is playing softly. Perhaps it does seep into her consciousness, for our aunt blinks, ever so slightly. She does so love that music!

5:10 p.m.

Your minutes are numbered, dear. Yours will be a calm passage. Those of us you leave behind are grateful that you are experiencing a "good death." Those years of anguish will soon be replaced by release and repose. As we watch you lie there, your soft white hair draped over the pillow, we see you are at peace, for you know you are not alone. You have your faith. You have your God. And we will keep our vigil until the very end.

5:11 p.m.

And now, Aunt Alma, we see the last vestige of color draining from your cheeks. You have only a minute or so more. Yet we can only reflect, this is a good death; this is a perfect death. Sharing this experience with you gives us an awareness of the deeper meaning of life in its closing hours.

5:12 p.m.

Gathering around a little closer, we, her family, while touching her hands, her shoulder, and drawing her as close to us as we can, repeat together our favorite prayer:

> Unto God's gracious mercy and protection
> we commit you. The Lord bless you and
> keep you. The Lord make his face shine
> upon you, and be gracious unto you. The
> Lord lift up his countenance upon you,
> and give you peace, both now and evermore.
>
> Amen

5:13 p.m.

Your time is here, Aunt Alma. You breathe heavily. A deep sigh. You take your final breath. Your heartbeat stops.
   It is over.

   Rest in peace, our beloved Aunt Alma. Your light perpetual will shine—will always shine, here in your home.

An old person loved is winter with flowers.
German proverb

Concluding Message to You, the Caring Family

Dear Friends,

To you who have lost a parent from this world, may I offer in loving support my empathy and my prayers, passing on to you a message that came when I needed it most?

> They are not dead who live
> In hearts they leave behind.
> In those whom they have blessed
> They live a life again,
> And shall live, through the years . . . and grow
> Each day more beautiful
> As time declares their good,
> Forgets the rest, and proves
> Their immortality.

Hugh Robert Orr

To those of you whose parent now resides in a geriatric facility, keep the faith, positive that you are doing the right thing. For now, at last, released from those uncertainties which once plagued you, you can garner your energies and use them wisely as, day by day, you demonstrate that Mother remains an integral part of your family.

Again I ask: Is she receiving good care to dignify her remaining years; is the care enabling her to retain her individuality and, to the extent possible, independence and control over her own life? With you, her "bulwark never failing," of course she is! And so, at this period of your life, may you be upheld by an inner peace—that peace of mind which you richly deserve, which you so painstakingly have earned.

Write to me. I care. Let me know how you are doing.

Sincerely,

Nancy Fox

Nancy Fox
1421 N.E. Eighth Street
Bend, Oregon 97701

Appendix

Skilled Care, Intermediate Care, Custodial Care—Defined

Skilled Care: Comprehensive planned care provided on an in-patient basis, requiring the supervision of skilled nursing personnel. This incorporates rehabilitation and restorative services, including such things as drug therapy, inhalation therapy, occupational therapy, or administration of intravenous fluids. The Skilled Nursing Facility is often abbreviated to SNF.

Intermediate Care: An intermediate-care facility is an institution licensed under state law to provide, on a regular basis, health-regulated care and services to persons who do not require the degree of care and treatment provided for in a hospital or skilled nursing facility. The intermediate facility provides care above the level of room and board, such as simple medical procedures, special diets, uncomplicated dressing changes and injections. Personal care is provided for by nursing assistants, licensed practical/vocational nurses, and, in some facilities, direct care is provided by registered nurses, as well.

Custodial Care: Care which provides assistance with personal needs such as meals, shelter, and assistance with dressing, etc. This care is provided for only by unskilled personnel.

Nursing Homes: How They Are Owned, Managed, and Regulated

Many homes are *nonprofit*, most of them under the auspices of the American Association of Homes for the Aging, 1050 Seventeenth Street N.W., Washington, DC 20036. These homes are run by church, government, or fraternal organizations at the federal, state, or local level. The vast majority of homes, however, are *for-profit* homes, in large part under the auspices of the American Health Care Association,

1200 Fifteenth Street N.W., Washington, DC 20005. Some homes are owned by individuals or corporations; many are part of a large chain of nursing homes.

The administrator is the person in charge of individual homes. He or she is licensed by the state, is appointed by the governing body, and is responsible to that body.

Nursing facilities must meet standards set by the state or local laws and regulations and must obtain a current state license or letter of approval from a licensing agency to operate. Those certified for Medicare and Medicaid must meet standards set by Federal regulations.

Homes are evaluated regularly by state agency surveyors or other public agencies to make sure that they meet health, safety, staffing, sanitation, and environmental standards, including the provisions of the Life Safety Code of the National Fire Protection Association.

Facts about Financing

Have a clear understanding about the financial aspects of your parent's stay in a nursing home. If you do not have your own lawyer, contact your local bar association. You may qualify for free assistance or be referred to a private attorney. If you have financial questions, contact National Senior Citizens' Law Center, 1709 West Eighth Street, Los Angeles, CA 90017.

Extra Charges: If a nursing facility charges extra for special services, keep a list of those you approve in advance—drugs, haircuts, personal laundry, etc. Both Medicare and Medicaid bar extra charges for such services as hand-feeding, wheelchairs, crutches, canes or walkers. Advance deposits on any special charges should not be required where Medicare and Medicaid are involved.

Spending Allowance: Under Medicaid, your parent is entitled to an allowance for personal expenses. If on social security, contact that office for information about their "representative payee" program to handle social security checks.

When Funds Are Exhausted: Will the nursing home allow the resident to stay there after his personal funds are exhausted and he needs Medicaid? If on a life-care contract, does the contract include medical care? Not all do. If your parent is eligible for Medicare and other insurance programs, contact your county department of social services, which can give useful help in planning.

How will Medicare or Blue Cross pay for the care needed? Just because a person is enrolled in a health-insurance program does not necessarily mean that nursing-home care will be paid for. Understand clearly how long the program will pay for such care, as well.

Self-Helps for the Stay-at-Home

Wheelchair Activities: A booklet by Arlene Gilbert—entitled *You Can Do It from a Wheelchair* (New Rochelle, NY: Arlington House)—covers meal preparation, floor care, laundry, child care, grooming, housekeeping, seeing the environment, special ways to put on clothes, and much more.

Equipment for the Handicapped: For a large selection of devices for walking, exercises, heat and cold therapy, furniture, massagers, armslings, safety devices, craft kits, etc., write to Preston Corporation, 71 Fifth Avenue, New York, NY 10003 for their catalogue. Also, write to Miles Kimball, Oshkosh, WI 54901, or Cleo Living Aids, 3957 Mayfield Road, Cleveland, OH 44121.

Model Bookmobile: A public library in Indiana offers a larger scope of services than most. A bookmobile with a wheelchair lift regularly visits five nursing homes, nutrition centers, churches, schools, clubs, and a county unit for the blind. It carries large-print books, talking books, and reading aids such as magnifying glasses, book holders, page turners, prism glasses, and reclining viewers. For more information, write to Supervisor, 815 Jackson Street, Anderson, IN 40616. Perhaps your local bookmobile could be expanded to include the above-mentioned aids.

Pamphlets and Catalogues

Home Health Care Catalogue: 48-page illustrated catalogue listing a variety of home-health products. Free at catalogue desk of your local Sears retail store, or write to: Home Health Care Catalogue, Sears, Roebuck & Co., Department 608, BSC8, 2 North La Salle, Chicago, IL 60612.

Products for People with Vision Problems: 160-page large print, illustrated catalogue listing hundreds of aids for people with vision problems. Free. Write to: Products for People with Vision Problems, American Foundation for the Blind, Dept. HA, Consumer Products Department, 15 West Sixteenth Street, New York, NY 10011.

Homecare Programs in Arthritis, A Manual for Patients: 23-page pamphlet offering exercise programs and ways to modify the surroundings for arthritis patients. Free. Write to: "Homecare Programs," Arthritis Foundation, Lennox Box 18888, Department AU, Atlanta, GA 30326.

Self-Help Manual for Arthritis Patients: 124-page illustrated catalogue listing hundreds of aids and homemaking tips. Send $1.50 to Self-Help Manual, Arthritis Foundation, Lennox Box 18888, Department AU, Atlanta, GA 30326.

Mealtime Manual for People with Disabilities & the Aging: 269-page illustrated catalogue listing hundreds of aids, homemaking tips, and purchase information. Write to: Mealtime Manual, Box 38, Ronks, PA 17572.

Special Books

Numerous free publications are issued by the Administration on Aging, U.S. Department of Health and Human Services, 330 Independence Avenue S.W., Washington, DC 20201, such as: *Are You Planning on Living the Rest of Your Life?* Write for their list.

Bibles in Braille: In addition to making the Bible available in many languages, the American Bible Society also provides Scripture on records, cassettes, and open-reel tape for the visually handicapped. When possible, some users give contributions to this cause, which makes it possible. Inquire at your local library.

Talking Books: Available through your public library. A doctor or qualified librarian will ascertain the need of the person making application.

Excellent publications are also available through centers that work with the aging. Write for their catalogues. These include:

Andrus Gerontology Center, University of Southern California, Los Angeles, CA 90007

New England Center for Gerontology, University of New Hampshire, 15 Garrison Street, Durham, NH 03824

Potentials Development for Health and Aging Services, Inc., 775 Main Street, Suite 325, Buffalo, NY 14203

Sister Kenny Institute, 2727 Chicago Avenue, Minneapolis, MN 55407

Recommended Reading

A Home Is Not a Home, by Janet Tulloch. Seabury Press, New York.

Aging: An Album of People Growing Old, by Shura Saul. John Wiley & Sons, Inc., New York.

Fantasy/Validation Therapy, by Naomi Feil. 4614 Prospect Avenue, Cleveland, OH 44103.

Green Winter: Celebrations of Old Age, by Elise Maclay. Reader's Digest Press. Distributed by McGraw-Hill Book Company.

How to Put JOY into Geriatric Care, by Nancy Fox. Geriatric Press, Inc., 1421 N.E. Eighth Street, Bend, OR 97701.

I Love You But You Drive Me Crazy: Guide for Caring Relatives, by Ann Calder and Jill Watt. Fforbez Enterprises, Inc., Box 35340, Vancouver, British Columbia, Canada V6M 4G6.

Living in a Nursing Home: A Complete Guide for Residents, Their Families and Friends, by Sarah Greene Burger and Martha D'Erasmo. Seabury Press, New York.

Ministry and Older People: Claiming a New Frontier, by Robert McClellan. A book to revitalize church life through ministry to, with, and for the aged. Andrus Center, University of Southern California, Los Angeles.

Nursing Homes: A Citizens' Action Guide, by Linda Horn and Elma Griesel. Beacon Press, Boston.

Ombudsman for Nursing Homes: Structure and Process. U.S. Department of Health and Human Services, Office of Human Development, Administration on Aging, Washington, DC 20201.

Report to the Congress of the United States, by the Comptroller General. *Entering a Nursing Home—Costly Implications for Medicaid and the Elderly.* Available through the U.S. General Accounting Office, Washington, DC 20548.

Special Problems in Long-Term Care: Documented Hearings of the Select Committee on Aging, House of Representatives, 96th Congress, October, 1979. U.S. Government publication #96-208.

The Other Generation Gap: The Middle-Aged and Their Aging Parents, by Dr. Stephen Z. Cohen and Bruce Michael Gans. Follett Publishers, Chicago.

Thirty Dirty Lies about Old, by Hugh Downs. Argus Communications, Niles, IL.

Working with the Aged: Practical Approaches in the Institution and in the Community, by Marcella Bakur Weiner, Albert J. Brok, and Alvin M. Snadowsky. Prentice-Hall, Inc., Englewood Cliffs, NJ.

Working with the Elderly: A Training Manual. Edited by Elizabeth S. Deichman and C. P. O'Kane. Potentials Development for Health and Aging Services, Inc., 775 Main Street, Suite 325, Buffalo, NY 14203.

Why Bother: He's Old and Confused, by Mary Judd. Winnipeg Municipal Hospital, Winnipeg, Manitoba, Canada R3L 2P4.

Nongovernmental Organizations Concerned with Nursing Home Affairs (partial list)

American Association of Homes for the Aging
1050 Seventeenth Street N.W., Suite 770
Washington, DC 20036

American Health Care Association
1200 Fifteenth Street, N.W.
Washington, DC 20005

American Association of Retired Persons
1909 K Street, N.W.
Washington, DC 20006

Gray Panthers
6342 Green Street
Philadelphia, PA 19144

Nader's Retired Professional Action Group
2000 P Street, N.W.
Washington, DC 20036

National Council on the Aging
1828 L Street, N.W.
Washington, DC 20026

National Council of Senior Citizens
1511 K Street, N.W.
Washington, DC 20005

National Senior Citizens' Law Center
1709 West Eighth Street
Los Angeles, CA 90017

Federal Government Agencies Concerned with Aging and Nursing Homes: Department of Health and Human Services

Executive Branch:

Office of Nursing Home Affairs
5600 Fisher's Lane, Room 17B-07
Rockville, MD 20852

Social Security Administration
Bureau of Health Insurance
601 Security Boulevard
Baltimore, MD 21235

> *Note:* Medicare-Medicaid eligibility and benefit information may be obtained from your local Social Security Office.

U.S. Administration on Aging
300 Independence Avenue, S.W.
Washington, DC 20201

> *Note:* Contact Director of Special Nursing Home Interests.

Legislative Branch:

U.S. Subcommittee on Aging
Subcommittee on Long-Term Care
Room 3121, Dirksen Senate Office Building
Washington, DC 20510

State Agencies Administering the Older Americans' Act

Alabama

Commission on Aging
740 Madison Avenue
Montgomery, AL 36104

Alaska

Department of Health
Office on Aging
Pouch H
Juneau, AK 99811

Arizona

Bureau on Aging
543 East McDowell
Room 217
Phoenix, AZ 85004

Arkansas

Office on Aging
Department of Social and
  Rehabilitation Services
Seventh and Gaines
Box 2179
Little Rock, AR 72202

California

Office on Aging
455 Capitol Mall
Suite 500
Sacramento, CA 95814

Colorado

Department of Social Services
1575 Sherman Street
Denver, CO 80203

Connecticut

Department on Aging
90 Washington Street
Room 312
Hartford, CT 06115

Delaware

Division of Aging
2413 Lancaster Avenue
Wilmington, DE 19805

District of Columbia

DC Office on Aging
1012 Fourteenth Street, N.W.
Suite 1106
Washington, DC 20005

Florida

Division of Aging
Department of Health
1323 Winewood Boulevard
Tallahassee, FL 32301

Georgia

Office of Aging
Department of Human
   Resources
47 Trinity Avenue
Atlanta, GA 30334

Guam

Office of Aging
P.O. Box 2816
Agana, Guam 96910

Hawaii

Commission on Aging
1149 Bethel Street
Room 311
Honolulu, HI 96813

Idaho

Idaho Office on Aging
Statehouse
Boise, ID 83720

Illinois

Department on Aging
2401 West Jefferson
Springfield, IL 62706

Indiana

Commission on Aging
Graphic Arts Building
215 North Senate Avenue
Indianapolis, IN 46202

Iowa

Commission on Aging
415 West Tenth Street
Jewitt Building
Des Moines, IA 50319

Kansas

Department of Social Services
State Office Building
Topeka, KS 66612

Kentucky

Aging Program Unit
Department of Human
   Resources
403 Wapping Street
Frankfort, KY 40601

Louisiana

Governor's Office
of Elderly Affairs
P.O. Box 80374
Baton Rouge, LA 70898

Maine

Office of Maine's Elderly
Department of Human
   Resources
State House
Augusta, ME 04330

Maryland

Office on Aging
State Office Building
301 West Preston
Baltimore, MD 21201

Massachusetts
Department of Elderly Affairs
120 Boylston Street
Boston, MA 02116

Michigan
Office of Services to the Elderly
3500 North Logan Street
Lansing, MI 48913

Minnesota
Governor's Citizens' Council
  on Aging
Suite 204
Metro Square Building
St. Paul, MN 55101

Mississippi
Council on Aging
802 North State Street
Jackson, MS 39201

Missouri
Department of Social Services
Box 570
Jefferson City, MO 65101

Montana
Department of Social Services
Box 1723
Helena, MT 59601

Nebraska
Commission on Aging
State House Station
300 South Seventeenth Street
Lincoln, NE 68509

Nevada
Division on Aging
Department of Human Services
201 South Fall Street
Nye Building
Carson City, NV 89701

New Hampshire
New Hampshire State Council
  on Aging
Box 786
Concord, NH 03301

New Jersey
Division on Aging
Box 2768
Trenton, NJ 08625

New Mexico
Commission on Aging
408 Galisteo Street
Villagra Building
Santa Fe, NM 87503

New York
New York State Office for
  the Aging
2 World Trade Center
Room 5036
New York, NY 10047

North Carolina
Governor's Council on Aging
Department of Human
  Resources
213 Hillsborough Street
Raleigh, NC 27603

North Dakota

Aging Services
Social Services Board of
　North Dakota
State Capitol Building
Bismarck, ND 58505

Ohio

Commission on Aging
34 North High Street
Columbus, OH 45215

Oklahoma

Special Unit on Aging
P.O. Box 25352
Capitol Station
Oklahoma City, OK 73125

Oregon

Department of Human
　Resources
Program on Aging
772 Commercial Street, S.E.
Salem, OR 97310

Pennsylvania

Office for the Aging
Department of Health
Room 540, P.O. Box 2675
Seventh and Forster Streets
Harrisburg, PA 17120

Puerto Rico

Gericulture Commission
P.O. Box 11697
Santurce, PR 00908

Rhode Island

Division on Aging
Department of Community
　Affairs
150 Washington Street
Providence, RI 02903

Samoa

Office of the Governor
Pago Pago
American Samoa 96799

South Carolina

Commission on Aging
915 Main Street
Columbia, SC 29201

South Dakota

Department of Social Services
State Office Building
Illinois Street
Pierre, SD 57501

Tennessee

Commission on Aging
Room 102 S/P Building
306 Gay Street
Nashville, TN 37201

Texas

Governor's Committee on
　Aging
P.O. Box 12786
Capitol Station
Austin, TX 78711

Utah

Office on Aging
Department of Social Service
345 South Sixth Street
Salt Lake City, UT 84102

Vermont

Agency on Human Services
State Office Building
Montpelier, VT 05602

Virginia

Office on Aging
830 East Main Street
Suite 950
Richmond, VA 23219

Virgin Islands

Commission on Aging
P.O. Box 539
Charlotte Amalie
St. Thomas
Virgin Islands 00801

Washington

Office on Aging
P.O. Box 1788 M.S.
Olympia, WA 98504

West Virginia

Commission on Aging
State Capitol
Charleston, WV 25305

Wisconsin

Division on Aging
1 West Wilson Street
Room 686
Madison, WI 55702

Wyoming

Department of Health
New State Office Building
West, Room 288
Cheyenne, WY 82002

About This Book

In *You, Your Parent, and the Nursing Home*, Nancy Fox writes from a unique triple vantage-point: (1) A direct-care nurse, she has worked in nursing facilities in many states, close to patient, staff, and family; (2) she is the daughter of parents whose combined nursing-home residency was twenty-five years; and (3) she herself has just "joined the club," i.e., reached the "senior citizen" mark.

Mrs. Fox knows the "good" nursing facility and will steer you to it. If your parent is already a resident, the author will define your role in supporting or bettering the care. She warns of the home where care is inadequate or the one to be shunned at all costs.

Her concern is for you, the family, whose feelings are seldom recognized, whose crucial role in the well-being of an institutionalized parent too often is untapped, ignored, or even discouraged.

Have you felt helpless, not knowing why? Not known what to expect, or where you fit into that formidable triangle made up of clients, staff, and administration? Now you will piece together the puzzle as you and the author take the Grand Tour of nursing facilities. What about that "nice" nursing home up the street? What goes on in there? Is it really just that—"nice"—or is it a disaster?

You will peek backstage both during and after visiting hours, by day or in the dead of night, to witness "inner sanctum" conditions, happenings, attitudes. You will learn what to observe, how to evaluate the care. Does your parent lead a meaningful life or is he/she simply being rolled down the conveyor belt of conformity? How can you, the family, become influential in bettering that care?

The goal is high. Total care for the total person, encompassing mind, body, and spirit. And then, gathering up your new insights, you will find that you *can* cope with your whole range of feelings, can channel that marvelous energy to constructive use.

Whether to place a parent in a nursing home is a difficult decision. But now, make that decision count, not only for your loved one, but for *you*. Nancy Fox is with you every step of the way. For it is only through you and your participation, she believes, that the American nursing home can approach the degree of excellence that the public—that is, *you*—have a right to expect.

www.ingramcontent.com/pod-product-compliance
Lightning Source LLC
Chambersburg PA
CBHW031249290426
44109CB00012B/499